PREVENTABLE

PREVENTABLE

THE INSIDE STORY
OF HOW LEADERSHIP
FAILURES, POLITICS, AND
SELFISHNESS DOOMED
THE U.S. CORONAVIRUS
RESPONSE

ANDY SLAVITT

St. Martin's Press
New York

First published in the United States by St. Martin's Press, an imprint of
St. Martin's Publishing Group

PREVENTABLE. Copyright © 2021 by Andy Slavitt. All rights reserved. Printed in the
United States of America. For information, address
St. Martin's Publishing Group, 120 Broadway, New York, NY 10271.

Design by Meryl Sussman Levavi

The Library of Congress Cataloging-in-Publication Data is available upon request.

ISBN 978-1-250-77016-5 (hardcover)
ISBN 978-1-250-77017-2 (ebook)

Our books may be purchased in bulk for promotional, educational, or business
use. Please contact your local bookseller or the Macmillan Corporate and
Premium Sales Department at 1-800-221-7945, extension 5442, or by email at
MacmillanSpecialMarkets@macmillan.com.

First Edition: 2021

1 3 5 7 9 10 8 6 4 2

To our career civil servants, who serve this nation with honor and skill, and to every health care worker who cared for us, who held a hand, cleaned a room, and absorbed our losses.

And to my wife, Lana, who has taught me how to work for what matters, all while giving me true happiness. She also helped create two wonderful humans, Caleb and Zachary. I hope we give them what my parents gave me.

CONTENTS

Preventable Timeline

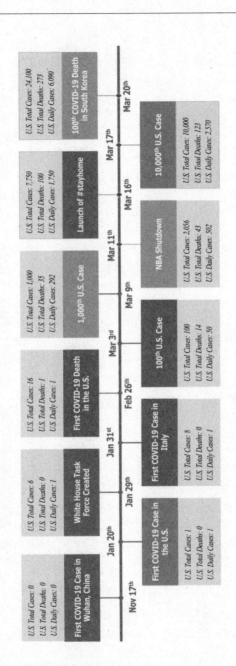

Preventable Timeline

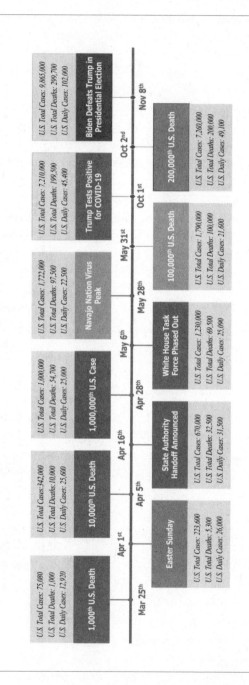

COVID-19 Data from covidtracking.com

PREFACE

In February of 2021, I was at my desk in the Old Executive Office Building, a couple of hundred yards from the West Wing. I was three weeks into my new role as White House senior advisor for the COVID-19 response and starting my fourth Zoom call of the day. Thousands of Americans were dying daily. The country was in desperate need of some good news after the yearlong pandemic.

A few minutes after the call started, my cell phone rang from an unlisted D.C. number. I hadn't been through an uninterrupted call in the last three weeks. I silenced it.

My phone rang again. This time I picked it up. It was the president's assistant asking if I could come to the Oval Office for a meeting already in progress. I grabbed a notebook and half-jogged to the Oval, where I found President Joe Biden, his chief of staff, Ron Klain, and Jeff Zients, the COVID-19 response czar, in the adjoining dining room. Biden motioned for me to join them at the table.

"Tell me what's going on in a way a junior in high school would understand it," he said to the three of us. The global pandemic had been gutting the country for the past year—upending and ending lives, shutting down businesses and causing job losses, and sparking a national identity crisis for a nation that considered itself above many of the world's problems. Biden's promise to the American people to lead us out of the pandemic was one of the reasons he was sitting there. Helping deliver on that promise was the reason I was there as well.

Ron, Jeff, and I told him that for many of the questions the public wanted answers to—like when the pandemic would be over— the answers were as yet unknowable. We had estimates, plans, and models, but that was all they were. And after a year of the Trump administration promising that the pandemic was about to end at any moment, the public had grown fatigued and distrustful.

"'We don't know' is a perfectly acceptable answer," the president said. "Let's give it to people straight." With nearly 500,000 American lives already lost—20 percent of the world's deaths from COVID-19, though we had only 4 percent of the world's population[1]—he said he wasn't interested in what made him look good, just straight facts he could communicate to the public. No games, just the truth.

This was another reason President Biden was sitting there; his sensibility was 180 degrees from that of his predecessor, Donald Trump. I had spent the past year watching the pandemic ravage the country from an unusual seat, on the phone with the Trump team, state officials, scientists, members of Congress, and others at the center of this storm, pushing for actions to improve our response to the crisis. I had become part-time helper, part-time critic, and full-time public chronicler. Seven years before, I'd had my own experience leading a large-scale national rescue effort, first from outside the government, then from inside it. I was one of the few people—and certainly one of the only Democrats—who was talking to the Trump White House on a regular basis during the first year of the pandemic, and I had developed a clear understanding of what was wrong with their response.

The White House in 2020 was not led by a man I respected or trusted. At the outset, that hadn't deterred me. After all, the color of your T-shirt shouldn't matter during a global pandemic.

But this was the White House of Donald J. Trump—a man whose ego wouldn't allow him to acknowledge a problem like the novel coronavirus emerging on his watch. All the things he would have needed to do—beginning with taking accountability, managing a large-scale response, calling for unity, and relying on experts and institutions of science—were anathema to him.

Still, I tried. I contacted Jared Kushner, the president's son-in-law and senior advisor, to offer my assistance, and spent the year on the push and pull of an effort to save lives and prevent even more colossal mistakes. Despite a few successes, when it came to dealing with the White House I generally found myself fighting the forces of denial, blame, and a short attention span that only blew more life into the pandemic. I put more energy into working with governors, mayors, private companies, and scientists—anyone who needed help or could lend a hand. I also began to publicly document what I was seeing every day—not just for myself, but for the public—in a nightly Twitter tweetstorm and in national publications that became a mainstay for many Americans seeking insight into what was happening. I made frequent TV appearances and started a podcast with my bright but bored 18-year-old son, Zach. My views were not formed by what I read in the paper, but from regular conversations with medical providers on the front lines and a whole host of people who would become principal players during the pandemic: people inside the Trump world like Anthony Fauci, Deborah Birx, and Kushner; governors in a dozen states; leading pandemic and scientific experts; and organizations that were central—or at least should have been—to defeating the pandemic.

I also began to write this book, which I came to call *Preventable*. This is a story full of missed opportunities, willful neglect, and indifference and denial from our president. But the country's experience during the pandemic is also a culmination of many of the things that had begun to distort our society for a number of years—gross inequality based on race and income, the growing distrust of expertise, a media addicted to promoting controversy, and a people long out of the habit of shared sacrifice for the common good. So many Americans did not have to die. Some of our mistakes could have been avoided had we had a different and better leader. Others were more deeply rooted in our American identity; those are more challenging to address and may be even more important to fix as we move forward.

This book is not meant to be full of sage commentary and policy prescriptions. Instead it follows the stories of some of the key people and events at the center of the crisis. Once you see what I saw, I think the lessons will emerge pretty much on their own. The solutions—well, that's another matter.

A few weeks after wrapping up the book, sometime between Christmas and New Year's Day, I received a call from the Biden team asking me to join the White House to help lead the pandemic response in the new administration. The crisis was raging and the newly authorized vaccine rollout was in trouble. Meanwhile, the normal transition of government was being hobbled by Trump's refusal to acknowledge the election results and his attempt to overturn them. Given the gravity of the challenge, I decided to say yes. It wasn't the first time I had been asked to help the country through a dire situation with an uncertain outcome. A quick digression will help explain how I came to be involved in this story.

■ ■ ■

In many ways, my career has been dominated by a series of blind leaps of faith. In 1998, I was five years out of Harvard Business School, newly married, and leading a charmed existence. In January, however, my college roommate and close friend, Jeff Yurkofsky, began experiencing numbness in his arm. We were both 31. He was soon diagnosed with inoperable brain cancer. Five months later, on July 2, he passed away, leaving behind not just his friends but his young wife, Lynn, and year-old twins, Josh and Judy. It wasn't actually what happened while Jeff was alive but what took place after he died that drove me to leave a fairly typical post-MBA career path and embark on what has become a decades-long journey to improve our system of health care.

Still in shock and struggling, Lynn moved with the twins across the country to live with my wife, Lana, and me and our new baby son, Caleb, in our California home. Wherever she went, medical debt collectors followed her. Jeff's fight for his life had meant costly medical care that wasn't always in-network or covered by his insurance. After many phone calls and appeals to hospitals, doctors, and labs, we helped her avoid bankruptcy, but only narrowly. And so in 1999, disturbed by Lynn's experience with medical debt, I started a business to help other uninsured and underinsured Americans avoid the same fate. This was well before the Affordable Care Act (ACA), also known as Obamacare, and in a time when uncovered health care expenses drove hundreds of thousands of Americans into personal bankruptcy every year.

Obamacare passed in 2010 with the promise to bring affordable health coverage to millions of Americans who had been left on the sidelines. In October 2013, however, the launch of its Healthcare.gov website publicly and spectacularly crashed, threatening to end Obamacare before it got started. Millions of Americans were in limbo. By this time I had worked in health care for over a decade, leading larger and larger health care organizations. So I cold-called the Obama administration and offered to bring a team to D.C. to help out. To my surprise, they accepted, most likely because they had no other offers.

On October 24, 2013, I traveled to D.C. to lead the rescue effort to save the health insurance exchanges, and the program itself. This was my second big leap into an unknown abyss, this time with health care for millions and a presidency itself at stake. My hope was to give Obamacare a fighting chance to close some of the major health care gaps that exist in our country. After five weeks of constant work and crisis management, our team managed to do the nearly impossible, and Obamacare was up and running. As the years passed, the value of that work became evident. By 2016, 20 million more Americans finally had access to health insurance—something that changed many people's lives for the better.

With Obamacare back on track, I took another leap and left

my job in corporate America to lead the Centers for Medicare and Medicaid Services, a federal agency responsible for overseeing the health care of more than 130 million Americans—most of them living on fixed or low incomes. I rented an apartment within walking distance of the Health and Human Services Department and commuted back and forth each week from Minneapolis, where Lana and I were living with our two teenage sons, Caleb and Zach. The work was tremendously fulfilling. Each day I had the opportunity to respond to people's problems and make decisions that improved the lives of millions of people. I also got a crash course in Washington 101, spending a significant amount of my time defending Obamacare in hearings held by a Republican-controlled Congress hell-bent on tearing it down.

In 2017, after Donald Trump became president and I left government, I envisioned returning home to a quiet, private existence. But when Trump and his allies in Congress made dismantling Obamacare a priority, I abandoned my plans and instead barnstormed the country rallying Americans to push their members of Congress to vote against repealing the law. I held town halls in red and purple districts, inviting Republican members of Congress who had voted in the past to repeal Obamacare to join me in hearing from their constituents. None of them ever did, but tens of thousands of their constituents showed up to share stories of how the ACA had improved their lives and ask what they could do to save it.

That spring and summer changed me. I became something of an outsider's insider—comfortable walking the halls of power in D.C., but with a growing understanding of how much power there was in the voice of the people and their stories.

■■■

This book benefited not only from what came before I wrote it, but (rather unusually) also what happened afterward. In early 2021, after submitting the final manuscript, working out of the White House every day, I got the rare opportunity to walk the same halls as the people I'd written about, and to ask myself how true my telling was. The publisher invited me to reread every word. Doing the work, after all, offers an entirely different perspective from seeing it from the outside. Now I was no longer in the cheap seats, but in the hot seat myself with a chance to see if I would need to eat any of my words. Would my perspective on the events of the first year look different once the weight of responsibility fell on my shoulders?

I was serving in a very different administration, led by a very different president. But I got a chance to see the scars and successes of our COVID-19 response from up close. I interacted with many of the people I had written about in this book. Many of the things I was most critical of the Trump administration for—not playing it straight with the American public, avoiding accountability, discarding science, playing politics, and ignoring the consequences of their actions in the lives lost—I was now on the hook for myself. And I became part of a team of people trying not only to defeat the pandemic but also to restore the parts of our government that had been decimated by the prior administration.

At first, I felt a deep weight of responsibility unlike anything I had ever felt before. By January 20, 2021, the first day of the new administration, people were dying by the thousands each day, new variants of the virus were emerging, and the vaccine rollout was a mess. But I also felt something different, something quite comforting: the presence of a committed president and people all around me in government who were competent and capable, and whom I could trust to go fast and respond with urgency.

All of these events led me to believe in the themes in this book even more strongly than when I first wrote it—both the huge missed opportunity to prevent such an enormous loss of life and the rays of hope that are there if we learn our lessons.

I hope that as you read this book, you will experience the roller coaster of what the first year of the pandemic felt like without the fear that was present at the time. And I hope it will spur in you a newfound commitment to resolving our country's biggest problems together with the many people who wake up every day and work on our behalf.

PREVENTABLE

INTRODUCTION

One day in April 2020, Ahmed Aden returned home from his warehouse job in Shakopee, Minnesota. He was shaking, sweating through his shirt, and coughing. He and his wife, Safia, feared the worst: for three weeks, Minnesota had been under a stay-at-home order due to the COVID-19 outbreak, but Ahmed was an essential worker and unable to work from home. At work, he was busier than ever, scanning and loading packages of necessities and diversions to be delivered to customers who were isolating at home.

For the next few weeks, Ahmed was confined to one of the two bedrooms in their apartment, while Safia squeezed in with their five children. Like a number of others with COVID-19, Ahmed couldn't afford medical care and, after two weeks, was no longer getting paid. In April 2020, no tests for COVID-19 were available for Ahmed or his family owing to a nationwide shortage, as well as a behind-the-scenes dispute between the state of Minnesota and test suppliers over how much money the suppliers would be paid. Despite working for Amazon, one of the world's most valuable companies, which was experiencing a huge surge in orders to make staying home more comfortable for its customers, without a test Ahmed didn't qualify for additional paid sick time.

Ahmed was isolated, but far from alone. Around the country, thousands and then millions of others found themselves in a similar boat, many in communities that were out of the public eye and which received little support when the virus hit.

■ ■ ■

About a month before Ahmed's infection, I sat in bed reviewing charts and emails from scientists who had an early understanding of how COVID-19 was spreading in Wuhan, China, and Lombardy, Italy. Their concern had grown, as had mine. Starting in February, I had gone on TV and written a piece for *USA Today* saying that the country needed to act quickly to avoid disaster. I was hardly the only one.

That day, March 12, the president downplayed the coronavirus entirely, as he had been doing for weeks, and assured the nation that "the virus will not have a chance against us."

I responded on Twitter: "This will be recorded as a major preventable public health disaster."[1] That tweet was viewed more than 10 million times (I'm trying not to say "went viral" anymore). As sometimes happens on social media, not everyone agreed.

There were only 50 Americans dead from the virus that day.[2] Within three months, 100,000 Americans would die.

March 2020 began a period unlike any the United States had ever seen. Unlike much of the world, Americans had almost no experience dealing with a public health crisis, and that left most of us, including our elected representatives in government, ill-equipped to confront one. As the White House tried to wish the virus away, Americans were left almost entirely on our own to prevent the damage from spiraling out of control. Even if we had started right away, it would have taken a number of weeks to slow the death toll and even longer for life to approach normalcy again. But the fact was, we weren't even starting.

With a highly contagious infectious disease, failing by even a little means that you get hurt a lot. And if you fail continually, the results can be tragic. Because COVID-19 is airborne, is highly contagious, and can be spread by people with no symptoms, the way it works defies intuition: its spread is not linear but exponential.[3] That's how 50 deaths on March 12 would become 100,000 by the end of May. It was like trying to swim after a speedboat that's 20 feet ahead of you. Even if you are swimming as fast as you can, every time you look up, it is farther away.

Over the coming days, I tried to do my part. I called on the best experts I could find and began an effort to urge the White House and state governors to act. Some did. Many didn't. I worked with teams of volunteers across the country to locate supplies for medical workers, help governors locate tests, and identify how to protect the populations that were most at risk. By the middle of March, I began to send a nightly report on Twitter to get facts out to a public awash in misinformation. These tweets attracted hundreds of thousands and occasionally millions of readers each night. Editors at *Medium* converted many of these daily reports into blog posts in order to reach more readers. As I learned specifics about different aspects of the pandemic—the acute shortage of tests and personal protective equipment (PPE), the tragic inroads the virus was making in communities on our tribal lands, what was happening behind the scenes inside the government—I shared it.

Over time, I learned just how many of the lives we lost and how much of the collateral damage we experienced could have been avoided. When COVID-19 reached our shores, we clearly weren't ready. As month after month went by and infections raged throughout the country, along with massive unemployment, business closings, and a significant rise in mental health challenges, we had a number of opportunities to reduce the damage. But we didn't take those opportunities.

Much of the blame clearly lands at the feet of Donald Trump; there, the inside story is both revealing and essential in establishing accountability. But, even accounting for Trump, other deep-seated issues that are part of our culture and national identity emerged to haunt us: Our obsession with individual liberties, even at the expense of others' lives and health. Our belief that the country can isolate itself from the rest of the world and rely on our wealth to protect us from global problems. Our increasingly unequal and separate nation, where people like Ahmed shoulder the lion's share of the risks and burdens. Our health care system, which is inaccessible to many even in normal times. Our diminishment of science and expertise.

Responding to a public health crisis requires decisive action, near unity, and a readiness to adapt as we learn about what causes the disease to spread and about what actions can effectively mitigate that spread. After his initial slow reaction, Trump had several chances to adapt and rally people to make simple sacrifices to reduce the death toll. But he did very little, and what he did, he didn't do very well. His sole decisive action—to shut down flights from China to the United States—was done in such a slipshod fashion that even after the official restriction was put in place, more than 40,000 Americans traveled from China to the United States, and screening was limited and spotty.[4] And, of course, he neglected to restrict travel from Europe to the United States for far too long.

The United States remained the global hot spot for COVID-19 even as growth in cases of the coronavirus in other parts of the world largely stabilized and then declined over the spring and summer. Months into the pandemic, basic resources and protective gear still weren't consistently available. Safe public health practices in use throughout the world, including mask-wearing, physical distancing, and contact tracing, not only were not implemented but also were openly scorned in many parts of the country. As things got worse, Trump moved to eliminate dissent inside the government and promised a series of silver bullets that he claimed would end the pandemic. All the while, he did not prepare, lead, or adapt; he did not even properly mourn our losses. When Trump himself was ill, he showed the same carelessness, putting those around him at risk and refusing to notify people he may have infected by not isolating early enough.

The cost of his failure, of *our* failure, was high. With only 4 percent of the world's population, the United States soon had 20 percent of the worldwide death toll.[5] To put it another way, by the end of 2020, we had lost more than the equivalent of a city the size of Cincinnati, Ohio. A response resembling what Germany and other developed countries mustered would have saved 70 to 80 percent of the lives we lost.

⋯

The United States had been spared global pandemics for far longer than most of the world. There are two types of defense systems when facing external threats like COVID-19: Our established defense procedures and the nation's ability to respond. When the United States' first line of defense against COVID-19—containment of the virus—failed, we were left to our own ability to react to minimize the damage. However, our society seemed unable to do what many other countries did—alter our own behavior enough to stifle the virus's ability to spread.

The continent of Africa is an interesting comparison. With nearly four times the population of the United States, Africa has suffered only a small fraction of the deaths due to COVID-19 as we have.[6] Africa doesn't have a particularly sophisticated first line of defense like the United States does. But African nations have long experience with infectious diseases and are able to mount a decent second line of defense when needed.

Our difficulty in beating back the pandemic shined a light on chronic issues that had been buried just beneath the surface for decades and whose costs suddenly became visible. Just as important as understanding why our government failed, *Preventable* looks at why our second line of defense failed. Minimizing the impact of COVID-19 isn't particularly complicated. Even as our government was underprepared and slow to move, we still had simple solutions at our fingertips, like wearing masks and temporarily avoiding larger indoor gatherings, that could have saved tens of thousands of lives, prevented millions from getting sick, and likely saved our economy from a prolonged recession. But we didn't use them.

In the United States, we have led a charmed existence, and we expect our wealth, our technology, and our self-image as an exceptional nation to keep us safe from the world's dangers without having to adapt our society. But the pandemic was not a test of our technology, our prowess, and our wealth; rather, it was a test of our political system, our health care system, our system of deregulated capitalism, our shared values, and our humanity.

Over the span of several generations, the United States has evolved from a country that sacrificed on a broad scale for its ideals and for the lives of others to one where a few months of isolation and wearing a mask was too much to ask. Hundreds, then thousands, of people began dying each day, often alone or in the presence of only a single nurse. Yet many citizens refused to respond to the carnage and discounted the fears of friends, neighbors, and family who were at risk, arguing that we should just move on. When the pandemic began, the United States was fractured along cultural, political, geographic, and racial lines. And when you're dealing with an infectious disease—particularly one that damages more marginalized populations while largely sparing better-off ones—even small cracks become huge fissures.

∎∎∎

Preventable goes inside the White House to show how much more could have and should have been done inside our government. Because our failure didn't begin and end with Donald Trump, or even start during his presidency, the book will also take you to the places in our country that have long been a single crisis away from devastation. And it will take you into the inner workings of our health care systems, our scientific agencies, businesses, and the media, showing how often their actions had a big impact—frequently for the worse.

This book is a fast "first draft of history" about the COVID-19 pandemic, but other challenges that offer little room for denial are already upon us or around the corner: antibiotic-resistant bacteria, the biodiversity crisis, climate change—and future pandemics. I will make the point in this book that we should view COVID-19 as our "starter bug." After all, the world is filled with viruses. With our charmed existence now shattered, we will see that COVID-19 will be recorded not as an overwhelming infectious disease but as one in which we overwhelmed ourselves. What if the next virus to hit our shores is seven times more infectious than COVID-19, like measles, and has a 70 percent fatality rate, like Ebola?[7] We simply must do better in the future—and this will require understanding why we have failed.

The first year of our pandemic response was unlike any other time in recent history. For all the needless death and suffering we have endured, the picture that emerges for me is not of a country that is hopeless but of a nation that must face its demons if we are to regain our potential for greatness and better protect our citizens against a coming wave of challenges.

Ahmed Aden and millions like him found themselves victims not only to a virus but also to a country that did not protect them and whose people abandoned one another. Our children and grandchildren will be the keepers of the story of this time period. All we can do is start at the beginning and take stock of what we let happen and what there is to learn.

CHAPTER 1

IS THIS REALLY HAPPENING?

Thia Morton, a 60-year-old documentary filmmaker, lived alone in her apartment in Vallejo, California, 30 miles north of San Francisco. On February 17, 2020, Thia had a cup of tea and went to sleep feeling fine. It was a Monday night, and she had a long week ahead helping care for an ailing friend. The next day she awoke feeling disoriented and had difficulty breathing. She had a low-grade fever and was barely able to drag herself out of bed. She made it to the bathroom just in time to vomit.

For the next three days, she was borderline unconscious, waking up and climbing out of bed only to make it the 20 feet to the bathroom to get sick; after that, she kept a bucket by her bedside. She had no appetite and lacked the energy even to get a cup of water. She thought of calling someone but found talking surprisingly difficult and painful. Two more days passed. She started having uncontrollable coughing fits. Her lungs sounded like crackling cellophane every time she took a breath. Then came horrible diarrhea.

A friend from Los Angeles called; hearing her rasping voice, the friend made her promise to see a doctor right away. Thia said she would, and fell back asleep. Mid-afternoon, Thia woke up in a cold sweat, her sheets soaked, and felt so bad that she dialed 911. The fire department and the EMTs arrived, and after their initial examination they radioed ahead to the emergency room team at Solano Medical Center that they were transporting a patient with an irregular heartbeat whose blood pressure was dropping.

When they brought her in, the nurse in the Solano emergency room saw that she was severely dehydrated and put her on an IV. Her blood pressure was 79/52, dangerously low and a sign that her organs were beginning to fail.

When the nurse mentioned the risk of organ failure, Thia asked, "Which organs?"

The nurse looked down at her and said, "All of them."

Later, when she had been rehydrated, she told the doctors she hadn't been to China, but that she was still hoping they could give her a COVID-19 test. At that point, however, the only tests available, those produced by the Centers for Disease Control and Prevention (CDC), were not working correctly. She tried to tell the doctors about her friend's daughter who had contracted some sort of flu while in Hawaii. She assumed they would ask about other people she had been in contact with and whom she might have infected, but no one did. After her condition was stabilized, she was sent home in a taxi, with instructions to follow up with her primary care doctor.

Though just 60, Thia had already had more than her share of medical problems. A rugby player, she had had six knee surgeries and seven concussions; she'd also suffered a near-fatal fall, had dislocated her kneecap giving birth, and had undergone a complete hysterectomy with complications. She was not soft—her parents, also avid rugby players, had brought her up to patch herself up and stay in the game until the final whistle blew. Still, the aftermath of her bout with COVID-19 has been the most challenging time of her life. Today Thia suffers from extreme exhaustion, shortness of breath, ongoing heart palpitations, a painful rash that extends from her neck to her eyeballs, edema, life-threatening blood clots in her legs and both lungs, and numbness on one side of her body from a mild stroke.

■■■

On February 24, just a few days after the EMTs rushed Thia to the emergency room, I appeared on MSNBC with Chris Matthews at the very end of a show that covered a host of topics, ranging from Michael Bloomberg's nondisclosure agreements to other politics of the day. When it was time for my segment, I tried to be as clear as I could: a pandemic was heading for the United States and the country was unprepared. President Trump, then in India, had been pressed earlier that day about the potential for an outbreak in the United States. "I think that whole situation will start working out," he said.[1] Of the 53 confirmed cases of coronavirus in the country at that point, he said, "They're all getting better." He knew better, as an interview with journalist Bob Woodward later revealed, though he would repeat versions of this even after millions of cases were diagnosed and more than 200,000 people had died.[2]

The Coming Storm

A few days prior, on February 20, 2020, I sat in my office on the fourth floor of a converted department store in the old Northeast neighborhood of Minneapolis, just across the Mississippi River from downtown. John Finnegan, dean of the University of Minnesota School of Public Health, was there to talk about starting a new program on politics and health care at the school.

As we made small talk, I asked Finnegan about the coronavirus outbreak in Wuhan, China. As the head of one of the leading public health schools in the country, and home to one of the leading centers on pandemic preparedness, I knew he would be privy to what was happening on the ground in Wuhan.

Wuhan is a major transportation hub for China—not the best place for an outbreak of an infectious disease. Finnegan took me through what they were seeing in Wuhan. Though the illness wasn't well understood, there was wide community spread already, meaning that people were getting the virus without knowingly coming in contact with a sick person. People were getting sick and being hospitalized at a record pace, straining the city's hospital capacity. More than 60,000 people had contracted the virus and 2,000 people were already dead, including doctors who had treated infected patients.[3] These events were first reported by the Centers for Disease Control to Health and Human Services secretary Alex Azar on January 3. Azar almost immediately briefed Trump's national security advisor, Robert O'Brien. And on January 25, Azar had briefed the president directly.

"What happens if it comes here?" I asked Finnegan, not yet aware of the extent that it already had.

"If it hits major U.S. cities, for many it will be a bad viral flu. But a lot of older people will need to be hospitalized," he said. One thing that caught my attention was when he said that, given what they were seeing in Wuhan, if COVID-19 came to the United States, "we could run short on ventilators."

I scratched the word *ventilator* down on a notepad. "Capacity? Who makes them? How fast can they be built?"

On Monday, March 9, I learned that a cruise ship filled with infected passengers had docked in Oakland, California. As I sat in my kitchen I reflected on a recent conversation I had had with Dr. Rhonda Medows, a senior executive at the largest hospital system in Seattle, where there was uncontrolled community spread. She was concerned that they were already experiencing shortages of just about everything they needed to treat COVID-19 patients.

I texted John Doerr to see if he was awake and could talk. John is a famous investor and has been a friend or mentor to just about every major technology CEO in the United States, including Steve Jobs, Andy Grove, Jeff Bezos, and Bill Gates. John and I were working together on a number of health care initiatives focused on helping underserved populations. John is also one of the country's leaders in addressing climate change and pandemic preparedness.

In that context, he had introduced me to many of the experts who were filling the gaps in my understanding of what was happening with the pandemic. At 69 and far from retired, John had the exacting mind of an engineer and the tenacity of an entrepreneur. He knew everyone, and he delighted in making connections.

Earlier that day he had emailed me two graphs, showing the progression of new cases in South Korea and Italy over the past few weeks. The South Korean progression was basically flat, indicating that the virus was under control. The Italian progression had started out flat and turned vertical very quickly, the result of exponential spread—that is, each infected person was infecting multiple people. The United States was two weeks behind Italy in the pandemic and had not yet experienced its level of case growth.

As John filled me in on the actions South Korea had taken—including large-scale testing and contact tracing protocols—I paced our front hallway. And then he said, "Andy, I'm afraid we are heading toward exactly the path that Italy is on." Italian hospitals were being overrun. The TV showed stories of desperate pleas from Italian doctors and ventilators being rationed while people lay dying in hospital hallways. Indeed, as Seth Doane, CBS's Rome correspondent, who had himself contracted COVID-19 in Italy around that time, would later recount to me about that crucial period, "One doctor told me, 'I wish we had locked things down 10 days earlier. . . .' So if you have people running around out there spreading, not really knowing, there's just that incredible ripple effect through communities."[4]

I asked John what we needed to do to get on South Korea's curve.

He hesitated before saying, "I'm afraid it's already too late."

More than even the words, his flat, dejected tone shook me. If the vertical line of case growth in Italy was applied to a country the size of America, that meant millions of cases, untold hospitalizations, untold deaths.[5]

At that point, we had just over 5,300 reported cases in the United States and not quite 80 deaths, mostly confined to a single state.[6] "Without testing," I asked John, "how do we even know that number is anywhere close?"

"We don't. It's a lot higher," he said.

We talked some more, and decided that drastic public action was necessary.

"Andy, why don't you go much more public about your concerns?" he asked.

I began to imagine the potential damage from a widespread pandemic. In addition to the disease itself, there would likely be massive job losses and business closures. Would society come to a standstill? And what about schools? Expecting something bad to happen and not quite knowing how to alert people, I felt a strange, almost adrenaline-like physical sensation—the kind of feeling you might get if you were watching a house fire start and knew there were people asleep inside.

Washington, D.C., 2013

The long days and sleepless nights of spring 2020 reminded me of the several months I had spent in 2013 living out of a hotel in Virginia and working 20-hour days on what felt like a life-or-death task: leading the turnaround of Healthcare.gov, whose disastrous rollout threatened Obamacare. Afterward, I was asked to join the administration to head the Centers for Medicare and Medicaid Services (CMS), where I oversaw health care programs affecting millions of Americans.

Those years in D.C. and my years in health care gave me a rare bird's-eye view of the highly complex U.S. health care system, which accounted for 18 percent of the U.S. economy and tens of millions of jobs.[7] Many Americans get a raw deal when it comes to health care. The system is highly variable, and even the parts that work well only work well for some people. Millions lack access to adequate health care, while a small number of large corporations make billions of dollars in profits.

My time in Washington opened me to a new world—one of

policies, politics, and politicians. The phone would ring all day long with senators and the White House and lobbyists on the line, each arguing for different things or calling me to hearings, and I was constantly making decisions that disappointed or pissed off powerful people. But trying to make health care better for millions of people on low or fixed incomes was an amazing responsibility, and I loved every minute of it. I began each day by reading emails from Medicare and Medicaid beneficiaries before heading into the office. No matter what the issue was, I responded with a personal note and follow-up, fully expecting they'd fall over in shock that a government bureaucrat wrote them back.

Setting Up Shop in Edina, Minnesota

Having led the country out of a different sort of health care crisis, I soon found myself at the center of the coronavirus storm. In late February and March 2020, throwing on a suit jacket and dress shirt with my sweatpants, I went on TV several times a week from my home in Minnesota to warn an unsuspecting public that we were entering a time that was going to be uniquely challenging and would require some sacrifice from all of us. I wasn't alone in seeing this, but as the federal government continued to deny the problem, I grew determined to act, and I gathered a small group of others to take matters into our own hands.

The country was caught flat-footed. Emergency rooms in major cities soon were flooded with highly contagious patients. Nurses and doctors had to treat patients suffering from this mysterious infectious bug without sufficient PPE to protect them. As John Finnegan had predicted, ventilators that helped patients breathe were in short supply. And ventilators weren't as big a problem as the shortages of doctors, nurses, and staff. Traveling nurses would be offered up to $10,000 a week plus expenses to work in the nation's outbreak spots.[8] Respiratory therapists were in even greater demand. We were running dangerously low on cotton testing swabs, testing chemicals, protective masks, gowns, face shields, and, most tragically, body bags. And what most people wanted to know was who was in charge of fixing it all.

One thing the country seemed to be doing right from the start was jumping into vaccine research, thanks to several teams of government scientists who worked together to break traditional barriers. On January 11, 2020, Anthony Fauci and his team at the National Institute of Allergy and Infectious Diseases (NIAID), part of the National Institutes of Health (NIH), downloaded a gene sequence of the virus posted by officials from China. A member of Fauci's team, Barney Graham, and Rick Bright, the head of the Biological Advanced Research and Development Authority (BARDA), a special unit that invests in vaccines in response to viral threats, had been investing in a new approach to vaccine development, one that relies on messenger RNA (mRNA), through a company called Moderna. By January 13, NIAID sent Moderna everything it needed to begin work on a vaccine.

Despite the quick action, we wouldn't know for some time whether a vaccine would work until it had been tested in tens of thousands of people. If it proved safe and effective, it would need to be manufactured in sufficient quantity. In the meantime, the country couldn't be put on endless hold. There was so much else that needed to happen. Nurses were going to need to work 18-hour shifts in an environment made especially difficult given the large number of infectious patients. Things we were short of—masks, ventilators, even swabs to conduct diagnostic tests—were not manufactured in significant quantities in the United States any longer, and overseas manufacturers were supplying other parts of the globe as well. Governors and mayors had to make decisions about which businesses and public spaces should remain open and how to implement modifications to everything from buildings to transportation. Because our own behavior was our best defense until a vaccine could be distributed, the public would need clear communication about how the virus was transmitted, what was safe, and what wasn't. Congress would need to provide financial support to American families and small businesses. There was a lot to do.

Soon I had a makeshift war room set up in my home office to try to help. Many people signed on to help and to lead various initiatives. The team at United States of Care—a nonprofit I had co-founded with my former senior advisor at CMS, Natalie Davis, to work on securing health care for every American—dove in to support the states and Congress. Andrew Stroup, a tech-savvy entrepreneur with ties to Asia and experience untangling supply chains, led an effort to find PPE. Dave Calouri, an investor based in New York, traveled to the White House to join the team procuring ventilators and other supplies. Racial justice advocate and organizer DeRay Mckesson built a portal for volunteering and to allow people to access mental health care and other services. My business partner Trevor Price launched an initiative in New York City to bring essential services to the most vulnerable New Yorkers, an approach we would introduce in other major cities.

Between those folks and a number of others, we tried to cover every base where help was needed. Before long we were locating masks for medical workers, finding diagnostic tests for states, locating ventilators, publishing data on where the risks were highest, advising states and Congress through a rapid-response system, and working with the White House to help hold off the worst of the crisis. In the early days, it almost never felt like enough; it was as if we were trying to put out a raging forest fire using just a couple of hoses.

There was a lot to do most days, particularly while the White House was doing precious little. If I needed to call a former ambassador to the United Nations to understand the funding mechanisms at the World Health Organization (WHO), I did. If I needed to talk to the CEO of a company that should be producing more PPE, I would. If I needed to talk to someone at the Federal Emergency Management Agency (FEMA) or the Food and Drug Administration (FDA), or to the head of vaccines at the WHO, I would. And if it became clear on any of these calls that a hospital in New York needed respiratory therapists, or the state of Massachusetts was running low on testing supplies, or New Orleans residents needed free telemedicine, I would hang up the phone and act that very minute.

I still had a note in my pocket about ventilators when Colorado governor Jared Polis called. He was one of several governors to tell me he'd seen an internal estimate suggesting that the state would need several thousand additional ventilators.

I called Medtronic, one of the world's largest manufacturers of ventilators, and got Geoff Martha, its CEO, on the phone.

"So, Geoff, how do we make 50,000 ventilators out of thin air?"

He explained it was a several-month process to make ventilators— if you could find the manufacturing capacity. He was expecting Trump would require other companies to dedicate manufacturing capacity to this project.

"I think he will eventually," I speculated. I had talked to people in the White House and knew they were weeks from even considering this.

Geoff decided he would put all the plans to build a Medtronic ventilator directly on the internet and offer to provide unlimited technical assistance to anyone who wanted to build them. He did so on March 30, and two manufacturers stepped up, agreeing to convert their manufacturing capacity. I connected Geoff to the supply chain team at the White House. Even if things went perfectly, though, we were eight weeks from having enough ventilators. We simply couldn't afford to be on Italy's curve for that long.

No single thing I worked on was about trying to solve the crisis wholesale. Far from it. Most of the time it was about moving something from A to B that could help get funding, make a hospital safer, break the logjam on stuck resources, or help someone on the front lines get their job done.

Drip, Drip, Drip, Splash

Because few living Americans had ever experienced a pandemic (and because the administration refused to tell us what it knew), it was hard for many to imagine how an event that was happening in China could affect us here. For many, the wake-up call came on

March 11. That evening, our younger son, Zach, a senior in high school, had a varsity basketball game to play. As games go, this one was important. The Blake Bears had made it to the sectional semi-finals, farther than the school had ever advanced before. Blake is a small private school that eschews sports recruiting (and, apparently, admitting tall kids), but after four years of playing together, the kids on his team were improbably beating bigger, more established teams. It felt a little like we were living in one of those corny sports movies that Cal and Zach and I had watched and rewatched their entire childhood.

That night we arrived at the school early and looked over at the cluster of seats where we had sat for all the games that season. A bunch of other parents were already there. Newly purchased hand sanitizer bottles in our pockets, we took seats four or five rows away from them—and everybody else.

"Come sit here," said the mom of one of Zach's teammates, nodding to seats right in front of her.

"Sorry, we're socially distancing," Lana said, awkwardly trying out the new language.

Blake came out strong and built a slight lead over a team no one had thought they could compete with. I felt my phone buzz several times, but I was trying not to blink, let alone pull out my phone, lest I miss some of the on-court action.

A few minutes later the same mom who had asked us to join them before the game shouted my name. She held up her phone, saying, "Andy, did you see that the NBA just suspended the season?"

The first domino had fallen. A professional sports league doesn't just walk away from hundreds of millions of dollars unless something is very wrong.

Blake won by nine points. Zach's school was one game from the state championship, but this would be their last game.

A thousand miles south in Dallas, the owner of the Mavericks, Mark Cuban, was also watching a basketball game from his usual seat at the end of the team bench. As someone handed him a phone and he saw the headline about the NBA shutting down, cameras captured his mouth opening in surprise and his body lurching back in his chair in reaction. It would become a meme for the moment when many of us realized the magnitude of what was happening.

Mark had developed an interest in health care policy, and we'd worked on a few projects together. Over the years I've found that Mark is usually a few steps ahead of most people. But he hadn't seen this coming.

"I was stunned," he told me later. "You know, before the game, I had a meeting with the players and the coaches in the locker room. And Luka [Doncic, the Mavericks' star player, who is from Slovenia] asked me what I thought the chances were that the season would be suspended or canceled. Because he had seen what was going on in Europe with his friends. And I was like 5, 10 percent at the outside. . . . And then, you know, halfway or whatever it is through the third quarter of that night, boom."[9]

The event that led to the NBA shutdown is a story unto itself. Rudy Gobert was a seven-foot-one Frenchman who played center for the Utah Jazz. Usually soft-spoken, Gobert was at a postgame press conference on March 9 when a reporter mentioned the growing panic around the coronavirus. At the end of the interview, Gobert, not known to be a rash guy, playfully touched every reporter's microphone and recorder on the table. Two days later, the Utah Jazz–Oklahoma City Thunder game was postponed when rumors started circulating that Gobert was ill. He soon confirmed that he had tested positive for coronavirus.[10]

I asked Mark about the impact of Gobert's positive test. He said the belief among his players had been that if you were under 30, "the chances of you catching it were slim. The chances of it having any severe impact were slim. And there's Rudy catching it after fooling around and pretending it didn't exist. And not only did he catch it, he was showing symptoms and he wasn't feeling so well. And so as guys talked around the NBA, it was like, look, this is not a good thing. We need to take it seriously."

That initial reaction—to make light of the virus and show you weren't scared—wasn't unique to Gobert. Rep. Matt Gaetz of

Florida wore a gas mask on the floor of the U.S. House of Representatives to mock those who were concerned about COVID-19.[11] A week later, one of his constituents was among the first Americans to die.[12] Several months later, Gaetz contracted it himself. Boris Johnson, the prime minister of England, boasted that he would not give up shaking hands due to this silly virus.[13] Three weeks later, he was in the hospital in the intensive care unit. In June, Herman Cain, the onetime presidential candidate, tweeted that he would not be wearing a mask to a Trump campaign event in Tulsa, Oklahoma.[14] He caught coronavirus and died.

We were like people who had never seen fire before and who wouldn't believe it was dangerous without sticking our hands in the flames first.

At home after the basketball game that night, I struggled to know what to say to Zach. He'd just experienced one of the high points of his life, but what should have come next had been brought to an abrupt halt. I needn't have worried, because he thought of something I hadn't considered. "Everyone is mad at Gobert for spreading the virus and shutting down the league," he said. "He may end up being the hero. I think Rudy Gobert may have just saved a lot of lives."

What Zach and I didn't know at that point was that Trump had been sitting on information about the virus's potential for damage for well over a month. If not for the NBA and Gobert, Trump might have kept the country from paying attention for even longer. One seven-foot-tall basketball player woke us up. But only the federal government had the infrastructure to respond. Inexplicably, the White House still wouldn't mobilize it.

I spent the next week on the phone with hospitals and with city and state government officials. On March 14, after a long day of calls, I sat down and did something unusual. I started writing what I had learned on Twitter in the form of a series of linked tweets (what some call a "thread").[15] In that thread, I reviewed what was happening in Italy, talked about the woeful state of testing in the United States, and encouraged the White House to continue to increase lab test capacity, something it should have started weeks before. To my surprise, more than 6.5 million people looked at the 15-tweet thread. It was the beginning of a pandemic ritual. From then on, very few evenings went by when I didn't provide a similar update. I decided there was no piece of information I learned that I would agree to keep confidential if it could help people. On many nights, millions of people got information about the pandemic from these threads.

A Lonely Death

In the spring of 2020, the early part of the pandemic was striking in what was missing: public grief. But beyond the fear most people felt and underneath the chaos, there was a deep and lonely sadness.

On March 23, the president of the Minnesota Timberwolves, Gersson Rosas, invited me to participate in a team call with the players, their agents, their parents, and the coaches. The players' parents had lots of questions; every myth about coronavirus had reached them, and they were frightened. They had reason to be. The Timberwolves' star player, Karl-Anthony Towns, 24, was on the call. His mother was in a coma with COVID-19. She had lupus, which made her condition especially dangerous. The team said a prayer for her. Three weeks later, after she seemed to be getting better, Karl's mom, Jackie, died at a hospital in Pennsylvania at just 58 years of age.[16]

We learned that John Bessler, the husband of our friend Senator Amy Klobuchar, was in the hospital with COVID-19 and needed assistance to breathe. Amy was not allowed in to see him and was only able to speak to him if someone held the phone up for him. She described COVID-19 as a lonely disease "where you can't visit the person you love. You can't be at their bedside. You can't even meet the people who are taking care of them. You can only talk to them on the phone. And it's just against everything that we've ever believed in for family and values and who we are as a country."[17] Fortunately, John recovered.

On April 9, my close college friend Rob Keil texted to let me know his father had just died from COVID-19 in a nursing home in New Jersey. Rob's father had been a big part of my life for a time. In college, whenever any of our parents would come to visit, we would get to have a nice meal at a grown-up restaurant. Rob and his brother, Dave, were from West Orange, New Jersey, but now lived in Northern California and Atlanta, respectively. Seventeen years before, when my dad passed away, Rob had flown to Los Angeles for his service. Don't let anyone ever tell you that those things aren't remembered. But with Rob and Dave's dad, there wouldn't even be a funeral. And they couldn't fly home to comfort their mother.

Gretchen Whitmer, the governor of Michigan, who publicly clashed with Trump, told me that she had lost three loved ones to COVID-19.[18] Michigan's lieutenant governor, Garlin Gilchrist II, later told me he'd lost 21 loved ones. And Peggy Flanagan, the lieutenant governor in my state, Minnesota, lost her brother. Everybody who lost someone used the same description: *a lonely death*.

■ ■ ■

Every morning I held my breath as I pieced together the data sent to me overnight and looked for any sign that the spread of the virus was abating. Other than that, I had few rituals. Lana and I had both our boys home, the first time in a while they'd been around at the same time. Both boys were due to graduate and were doing their final semesters of school online. Caleb was about to graduate from college and, he hoped, find a job. Instead he was confined to our basement briefly after testing positive for COVID-19, which he'd been exposed to at school. While he waited, we brought him book after book. Zach was waiting to hear what colleges might be interested in admitting him. Both of them were missing a lot, and while we were a close foursome, this was not where they wanted to be right now. But their loss was Lana's and my gain, as having the four of us home, cooking together, eating together, playing ping-pong and pickleball, and watching movies together, was found time.

Like everyone else, Lana and I had had plans for 2020 that didn't include the pandemic. In addition to the two graduations, we'd had a summer trip planned to, of all places, China. Cal was looking forward to a successful job search and joining the world of college graduates in New York. Lana's sister, Lisa, was planning a late summer wedding. My sister, Lesley, and her partner, Doug, were building a house in Michigan we hoped to visit. My mom had a big birthday coming up that we planned to celebrate with a trip. Lana was leading the Minnesota elections team for the gun-safety advocacy group Moms Demand Action, and on top of the presidential election, there were a number of state and local contests she was focused on winning. And our empty-nest plan was to move to California, where Lana grew up, where we married, and where our kids were born. Besides all of that, at the end of January, my business partners at Town Hall Ventures, Trevor Price and David Whelan, and I had just launched our second fund, an unusual effort to invest in health care businesses serving low-income and underserved communities.

It soon dawned on me that all those plans—all of them, including getting up and going to work in the morning—were going to be upended.

We made the most we could of the time together. Zach and I launched what turned into a popular podcast called *In the Bubble with Andy Slavitt*, broadcasting twice per week and interviewing on-air some of the experts and politicians I regularly talked with.[19] The goal of the podcast was to provide a practical source of information, but also a warm and helpful guidepost for families. I pictured Winston Churchill talking to Britons in the toughest of times. I pictured Fred Rogers talking about love in a world of trauma. I settled on that Churchill-Rogers ethos to guide the show, plus a bunch of dad jokes I was sure people couldn't live without.

The complete truth is that I was also motivated by the fact that my 18-year-old son wanted to do something together—even if it was entirely the result of limited options. He soon became my monotone but heartwarming sidekick on the show, delivering "Zach's Facts" about COVID-19. If anything, I think we gave people a small sense of normalcy and hope when people were at their darkest and most uncertain. I'm grateful Zach stuck with it until it was time for college to begin.

We have had a lot of great people on the show: Tina Fey talking about life in New York, Ron Klain explaining how disaster response works, chef José Andrés on feeding people in crisis, people who'd invented new virus tests, administrators running school districts, NBA coaches on working within pro basketball's bubble, and an array of governors and senators. Still, one of the highlights was when I called my mom in her apartment in Chicago.[20] She was used to walking seven miles a day around the South Loop area of Chicago. Now, like many people, she was stuck in her apartment all day by herself. But she wouldn't complain. In fact, she was funny. "I want to say that out of every negative comes something positive," she deadpanned. "I'm gonna learn how to use the internet a lot better than I was able to before." It turned out to be true—we had Zoom cocktail parties with her during the months when we couldn't see her. I hope to have her humor and equanimity when I get to be her age.

The Novel Virus

That spring, as I gathered information and talked with hundreds of people, a picture began to emerge of the villain we were squaring off against. And it was a virus that baffled us.

COVID-19 was a particularly confounding infectious disease, which made it a particularly difficult challenge from the perspective of policy and public response. The virus spread surreptitiously from unsuspecting carrier to unsuspecting carrier. These carriers were often young and the virus often barely left a sign of illness in them, if it left one at all.[21] Superspreaders, a small portion of people who contracted COVID-19, could spread the virus incredibly efficiently—sometimes to thousands of people—while never being aware they had it.[22] We didn't know who these superspreaders were, but there were some estimates that 10–20 percent of those infected accounted for 80 percent of the spread.[23]

The virus could be dangerous for anybody without built-in immunity, but when it found someone with a weak or aging immune system, it was especially so.[24] It could spread through crowds, then lie quiet for days while it worked its way into the lungs, and through the lungs into the blood vessels, where it could go anywhere the blood traveled—the kidneys, the brain, the gut, the limbs, the heart, the pancreas—often fooling the immune system into overreacting.[25] Sometimes it would do its damage to the organ systems unnoticed. Sometimes it would kill people. While older and sicker people were at highest risk, it could cause mysterious but harmful symptoms in some young people too.[26]

When the virus found a friendly environment—one with a lot of people in close contact, sharing the same air, especially if there was lots of laughing, singing, or loud talking—it could do maximum damage.[27] The period before symptoms showed up, if they showed up at all, made the virus especially confounding to control. Unlike with the flu, contagious people with the coronavirus circulated much more freely. The places hardest hit were nursing homes, meat processing plants, detention centers, homeless shelters, crowded bars, church choirs, cruise ships, farm labor camps, and housing with multigenerational families. One person could infect dozens at a time. And anyone who came in and out of those areas—prison guards, nursing home workers who rotated between facilities before they knew they were infected, family members—could both bring the virus in and spread it back to the world beyond them.

If the virus was spreading in a community, it was hard to keep any place safe. Deborah Birx, the White House COVID Task Force coordinator, told me that nursing homes and communal settings couldn't be isolated from infections in the community. "The infections aren't a function of the quality of these institutions. They're a function of the spread in a community," she said. A study by the University of Chicago backed that up.[28]

Birx's point was important. You can't operate nursing homes without staff from the community, or prisons without prison guards. All these people have families, and all these family members go to work or school. If there is spread in a community and if places like bars, where the virus is transmitted easily, are open, the virus will eventually spread to all corners of the community.

As my friend and former FDA commissioner Rob Califf told me bluntly in his Carolina drawl, "This virus is aiming to thin the herd of the old, the poor, and the sick."

Anthony Fauci referred to the virus as his worst nightmare, given how it spread, how lethal it could be, and how it preyed on people.[29] Not only was there no vaccine, but at the beginning there were no good medicines to treat it either.

After several near misses with other deadly viruses in the United States over the last few decades, including Ebola, COVID-19 had become the virus of the century. Mass death, fear, uncertainty, and job loss were spreading rapidly along with the virus. But we weren't living in a "new normal" as much as we were waking up to an "old normal" that had existed around the globe for centuries. As some countries had already done and others were now doing, our nation would have to decide if we were going to get good at public health.

Voices in the Wilderness

I ran into Dr. Michael Osterholm at a Minneapolis television studio on March 15—the last time I did a broadcast away from home, as it turned out. Mike had published a book in 2017 about the near certainty of a global pandemic, calling out a SARS-like illness from China as a distinct scenario.[30] One of the world's leading pandemic experts, Mike oversaw the well-regarded Center for Infectious Disease

Research and Policy (CIDRAP) at the University of Minnesota. Over the years, many people felt that every day that passed without a pandemic seemed to be mounting evidence that he was engaging in needless fearmongering. Now, though, Mike was deeply worried, and he came across on television as dark and pessimistic. In person, he was an earnest, friendly midwesterner with a big smile and a gracious attitude. But Mike was also a realist who knew what lay ahead for the country. I found him fact-based to a fault and deeply knowledgeable about the subtleties of how to manage outbreaks.

On January 20, Mike had published a message on the CIDRAP website saying that a pandemic would soon overwhelm U.S. cities.[31] He projected that if the death rate stayed the same as the original rate in Wuhan, 800,000 Americans could die.[32] But even when an actual pandemic emerged and began to wipe out hundreds of thousands of people in the United States, critics still dismissed his warnings as something they didn't want to hear.

"We're in for an 18-month war. I don't think people realize the scope of this, Andy," he said to me as we stood in the hallway in front of the TV studio I had just exited and he was about to enter.

I asked him about the potential for a ventilator shortage and whether that meant that all Americans should be under a strict stay-at-home order.

"Not everywhere at once," he cautioned. "That will never work. Studies have shown people will listen to you for about two weeks, but if they don't see what you're telling them, they will begin to rebel. And they might rebel at exactly the time that the virus comes to their location. This is a very big country. You've got to manage this regionally and balance people's needs with the best public health response. More people will die, but that's the only way things will work." That got my attention. There was so much he knew that we would all be learning about soon.

Mike was about a foot away from me as we were talking. I felt a little funny backing away from one of the country's leading pandemic experts, but I did, and I asked him why he wasn't socially distancing.

"Look, the six feet means absolutely nothing," he said, referring to the social distancing norm that was being widely recommended. "You and I were in the same greenroom just now getting makeup right after each other. If one of us has it, the other one does. The virus aerosolizes." Aerosolization, which makes indoor spaces especially dangerous, was something that wouldn't really be in the public discourse for a number of months yet. Throughout the pandemic, Mike was about two steps ahead of the CDC and WHO.

The next time we were face-to-face, which wouldn't be until August, when we met with Deborah Birx, we were both masked up, and he kept his distance.

Mike was one of a number of people who had been warning in the early days of the pandemic about these unlikely-seeming events. So were Bill Gates; Bill Joy, the co-founder of Sun Microsystems; the Pulitzer Prize–winning journalist Laurie Garrett; and Larry Brilliant, the epidemiologist who was part of the successful effort to eradicate smallpox. They were the Cassandras of our era. Cassandra is a character from Greek mythology who continually warns of impending doom and whom people refuse to believe. When a Cassandra sits next to you at a dinner party, you will hear predictions of stock market crashes, hyperinflation, housing market crashes, asteroids hitting the earth, nuclear accidents, 100-year storms, massive computer viruses, or global pandemics. After an hour you will beg the host to move you to a different seat. Did these Cassandras expect us to plan for every possible event? Think about these unpleasant things? Live our lives as if there were a sword hanging over our heads?

The Cassandras were now warning us again, even if many people would still ignore them. Mike predicted that without a vaccine, up to 60 percent of us would be infected before all was said and done.[33] Other experts were saying that anywhere from 20 to 60 percent of the population would be infected.[34] The number of deaths they estimated in the United States alone ranged between half a million and 2 million. I didn't doubt that range was possible, but it's important to note that these estimates didn't account for improvements in care and for preventive actions we could take. But even when cutting those numbers in half, that meant hundreds of thousands of people in the United States would be dying—a chilling figure. Those were the stakes and what we had to wake ourselves up to.

"These numbers are not our destiny," I tweeted and wrote and said on TV whenever I got asked about these estimates. We were able to influence the outcome; we had to learn how. No matter how bad things got, I would continue to remind myself, we could always *save the next life.*

In many parts of the world, the people making these predictions would not have been considered Cassandras; they would have been seen more like weather forecasters on the news. But predictions of loss didn't seem real to Americans. Weather forecasters had been "wrong" before. And other countries had managed the SARS virus. Why couldn't we manage COVID-19? At first that was an honest, hopeful inquiry; later it became an expression of frustration.

One reason the United States has been so reluctant to prepare for and react to COVID-19 relates to the privileged existence we've led. The world is filled with infectious diseases. There are 10 other known outbreaks going on globally at the same time as COVID-19.[35] Many of them are contained to a single country or several contiguous countries. In the last decade thousands of people have died from widespread infectious diseases such as H1N1 and other influenzas, cholera, Ebola, measles, and dengue fever.[36] With the exception of the annual flu and HIV, the United States has largely been unscathed by such diseases in recent history. Ocean borders, first-rate disease control, and early warning systems had been successful enough that for most Americans, it took a while for what was happening in early 2020 to register. Even after it did, many were tempted to wish it away rather than accept their part in controlling it.

Other parts of the world were also taken by surprise by COVID-19 but reacted quickly. One of them, Hong Kong, had more cross-border traffic with China than any other territory. It has a direct train and direct flights to Wuhan and is one of the most densely populated cities in the world, with completely packed commuter trains. Yet Hong Kong didn't see its 100th death until September 12 and remains one of the least affected parts of the world (as of this writing at least).[37] Hong Kong had two important weapons the United States didn't: pandemic experience and the will to act collectively. The city of 7 million had been through a flu outbreak in 1968 that ended up killing 1 million people worldwide, and they'd been through SARS in 2003. Even though the new Chinese government in Hong Kong didn't begin its own response quickly and was not widely trusted, most people began wearing masks—without a mandate—by the end of January.[38]

They saw the same fire we saw, but they knew better than to touch it.

New York

Fifteen minutes after my conversation with Mike Osterholm, the car dropped me off at our home in Edina. I stood on our lawn in the cold and took a minute to look up into the dark Minnesota sky. It was so still that I could feel my heart beating. Was this threat real? It was hard to conceptualize. What could we compare it to? Would we soon be seeing scenes in hospitals we'd only seen overseas during wartime?

I walked into the house to find that everyone was asleep. I had a drink and reviewed emails and texts, and then tried to get some sleep. I couldn't. One message I had was from Rob Bennett, a progressive New York advocate and social media organizer. I had been reviewing graphs New York governor Andrew Cuomo was using to estimate case counts and hospital capacity. The graphs showed that if something didn't change rapidly in New York, their hospitals would be completely overrun and out of hospital beds and ventilators. Other governors, including in Kentucky, New Jersey, and Colorado, told me of very similar concerns. Rob told me that

Corey Johnson, the Speaker of the New York City Council, had reached out to him asking for my advice.

"Close the fucking bars," I texted Rob, displaying my usual subtle mastery of the English language. "Read the reports from Italy. It's what Italy wishes it had done. Those charts will only be the future for so long." I believed there was still time, but barely. "It's not destiny," I added.

Around one in the morning—2:00 a.m. New York time—Corey texted me: "Hi Andy, I'm so concerned. The tsunami feels near and NYC isn't acting drastically."

I suggested he share Cuomo's graphs with the public. Perhaps those would make it clear that half-measures would not be enough.

I reminded him what Mike Leavitt, the secretary of Health and Human Services under George W. Bush, had said: Every action taken before an epidemic looks like overkill. Everything afterward looks pathetic.

"We are dead on with Italy's curve," my text continued. "Only dramatic action in a place like NY changes things."

I sent a litany of recommendations, ranging from temporarily stopping all elective surgeries immediately at New York City hospitals and closing the airports to—most important—closing bars and restaurants.

New York mayor Bill de Blasio was still encouraging people to go out and enjoy themselves at restaurants, providing a field day for the virus. And—unlike in Hong Kong and other world cities—bars and restaurants in New York were still packed. Corey had been outspoken in calling for all nonessential services like bars and restaurants to be shut down.

While Trump was silent and de Blasio was encouraging social gatherings, Mayor London Breed of San Francisco, a first-term mayor of a city every bit as international as New York, declared a state of emergency at the end of February, aggressively calling for social distancing and banning large gatherings. In what was perhaps the closest U.S. parallel to Hong Kong, San Francisco had

had experience with a real public health crisis and infrastructure decades earlier, as it dealt with the AIDS epidemic.

The impact of New York's delay was significant. Both New York State and California hit 100 confirmed cases on March 8. California quickly issued a stay-at-home order, adopted social distancing measures, issued guidelines against large gatherings—including in bars and restaurants—and prepared to use hotels as quarantine facilities. New York took just six days longer than California to put similar measures in place.[39] By early April, New York hit 100,000 cases before California hit 10,000.[40]

At the time I talked to Corey, there were just over 5,300 confirmed cases in the United States and there had been only 90 deaths, but Corey understood something that was very hard to see: the power of exponential math.[41]

Zach's Math

Since the virus was spreading exponentially instead of linearly, a two-day delay in action could put you a month behind in containing the virus. The reason is exponential math. To go back to my swimmer-and-boat analogy: if you're trying to swim to a moving speedboat that starts out 15 feet away from you, by the time you swim those 15 feet, the boat could be 100 or more feet away.

The person I knew with the strongest qualifications on this topic was my 18-year-old son, Zach. He was something most of the rest of us were not: a high school math student. We were watching pandemic news coverage one March day when the TV anchor led with the usual news that there were a record number of cases that day. Zach had picked up on the tone of drama in the anchor's voice as he announced the climbing number of deaths each day.

"Dad, don't people understand how exponential math works?"

"Most adults don't naturally think that way, Zach," I replied. But that gave me an idea: a high school math word problem.

"Zach, what happens if one person infects 2.3 people? How many people would be infected after 10 generations of infections?" At that time, 2.3 was the average infection rate (R0), meaning that on average each infected person spread the virus to 2.3 other people. A generation was each set of newly infected people. With COVID-19, it was generally thought to take an average of five days between generations.

He entered some numbers on his phone and came up with the answer: 4,142. In other words, over the course of approximately 50 days, one person who had the virus could be responsible for its spread to more than 4,000 people. I was a little shocked.

"Wow. Okay. What if the infection rate was reduced from 2.3 to 1.3? Then how many people would be infected after 10 generations?"

His answer: 13.8.

I was in disbelief. "That can't be. At an R0 of 2.3, one person could infect more than 4,000 people in less than two months' time, but if the R0 was reduced by 1, only 14 would be infected?"

He nodded.

"What if it were 3.3?"

He did some more calculations. "A total of 153,158," he told me. That's a fast speedboat.

"That can't be right," I said, and made him do it again. He looked at me as if he was wondering whether I had ever attended school.

I looked up the estimated death rate, the percentage of infected people who would die. It was estimated at 1.3 percent at the time.[42] Later in the pandemic it would drop to about half that, due primarily to the discovery of a steroid treatment and better assistive oxygen procedures.

"So let's take an asymptomatic person with COVID. They could walk out of their house, and if they don't take any precautions, they could be responsible for 4,100 infections without even knowing it? At a death rate of 1 percent, that's 41 lives lost. Just from one unknowing person."

Zach nodded.

"Let's say one of your irresponsible friends goes out into a big crowd of people at a party and infects a lot of people, and they are all equally irresponsible. They could be responsible for 150,000 cases and 1,500 people dying. On the other hand, if your very responsible friends stay home and are much more careful, keep some distance from people, then 14 people end up infected. And nobody dies."

"That's a good way to talk about this. I think that will help people understand exponential math," Zach said to me. Finally, some hard-earned approval.

(Not long afterward, an "expert" challenged me to provide a source for the analysis that one person could transmit the virus to 4,100 people at the average transmission rate.[43] Zach suggested I reply with "Source: high school math.")

I thought about John Doerr's challenge to me to communicate to the public what was happening. Not only was the president not issuing warnings, but he was calling the virus a "hoax" and claiming that it would just disappear.[44] I hoped Mike Osterholm's gloomy estimates of 800,000 deaths turned out to be wrong, but the disease was most certainly not a hoax. I needed a way to communicate that would help people understand that the pandemic was very real, but I also wanted to avoid talking about numbers that would numb people, like hundreds of thousands or millions of potential deaths. People were already concerned, skeptical, and confused, and the exponential math that made these numbers possible wasn't intuitive. I realized that talking about COVID-19 as one individual speaking to another was perhaps the most effective way to convey information. It also had another benefit—which was to remind people that their individual actions mattered, a lot. That, without a vaccine yet, we were our best solution.

On March 29, at the end of a seven-minute interview on MSNBC with Kasie Hunt in which we talked about the large and accelerating number of cases and deaths, I tried this approach.

"What we have in front of us is an opportunity. Unlike prior generations, my generation has never been called on to sacrifice. We didn't go through the Rosie the Riveter era, and I realize for a great many Americans, being asked to stay home, losing precious dollars in their savings, having their kids miss important things in their lives, and being uncertain about the future is not a lot of fun. I don't want to take that for granted. But what if I could say that by doing that, you knew you could save 40 people's lives, which is about the calculation if you unknowingly infect someone? I don't know a person in the world who wouldn't do that."[45]

I could only gauge one person's reaction at the time, and that was Hunt's. Sitting in her home office, she managed a smile—rare for the moment. She went off script and talked about raising her own son while trying to bring us the news. And then she said, "I really appreciate your optimistic but sobering, pragmatic, and straightforward way of approaching this subject." It was exactly what I needed.

Save the Next Life

During those early days of the pandemic, I often reminded myself that I was living through history. And what feels messy and uncertain will someday look neat and tidy, with a beginning, middle, and end. Every day I received dozens of messages expressing anguish, sadness, loss, and uncertainty. Far from bringing me to grief, though, those messages had a way of keeping me calm and giving me purpose. These were meaningful times, I told myself. I imagined people in the future looking back on our response to the coronavirus. What questions would they ask? How would this all be evaluated? How would *we* be evaluated?

It felt like history would judge us on two things. The first was obvious: How many people did we lose, and how many of those losses could have been prevented? We would live with that judgment of history for as long as we were worth remembering. Whether the number was 10,000, 100,000, or 1 million, that would make the first paragraph on Wikipedia. The one thing that kept me going even when the country had a really bad day was the idea that *the next life could be saved.*

The second thing we would need to answer for was far more personal: *What did I do to help during the difficult times?* Most of us might not make the history books, but that question would be part of the oral history of the times, and the answer to it could have a lot to do with what kind of country emerged after the pandemic. The pandemic meant people hurting everywhere, people in need, people unsure how to put food on the table, people dying alone hooked up to tubes. To what extent would we overcome our own fears and offer help to people who needed it? The Fred Rogers line that when you're scared you should "look for the helpers" had never seemed more appropriate.

Save the next life. No matter what has happened before, every day the pandemic creates a new opportunity.

There is a counterargument that must be looked at. There are still some who believe that, given all the costs of fighting the pandemic, the country overreacted to the coronavirus crisis. Did they have a point? There's no denying that the pandemic and response felt different depending on where you were sitting. Who did you know more of—people who lost their lives or people who lost their businesses? And where do you place the blame?

CHAPTER 2

UNEXPLODED BOMBS

Scene: The years leading up to the pandemic

Before we jump into the events of 2020, it's worth a quick look at some of the things that allowed the United States' response to COVID-19 to go not just badly but spectacularly wrong. Several things that were failing us in normal times became significant impediments when we faced once-in-a-century events. It starts with a health care system that doesn't work for so many of us in an increasingly unequal society and extends to our priorities, our government, and how we have come to treat one another.

The United States' health care system is especially hard to explain to people living in countries that provide universal health coverage. Our system requires that people earn their care—either through their jobs, their income, or their age. Even then, our system has financial gaps, resulting from high deductibles, high co-payments, claim denials, and premiums many can't afford. Many Americans still lack insurance coverage, and most others still worry that if someone in their family gets really sick, they may not be able to afford to care for them.

Inequality in Health Care:
The Peloton Crowd Versus the Take-the-Bus Crowd

One of the most significant distortions in our health care system is its gross inequities. When I give speeches about our health care system, I discuss this problem in overly broad terms, but it gets the point across. I talk about a health care system that has divided us roughly in half. Half the people have employer-based insurance or are financially well-off enough not to have to worry about daily medical expenses.[1] They have enough money, relatively speaking, to be able to look after their health. They may need to lose a few pounds or lower their blood pressure a bit, but they are generally healthy, and they sometimes have a hard time understanding why everyone can't do the things necessary to keep healthy. I refer to this group (usually my audience) as the "Peloton crowd," after the nifty but expensive home exercise equipment whose ads promise a road to self-actualization—or at least to eliminating the 10 extra pounds your spouse frowns on.

The Peloton crowd does okay with the existing U.S. health care system. Even though they don't love it, they have learned how to navigate it and have good access to the doctors and hospitals they want when they get sick. They enjoy advantages like big provider networks, the advocacy of their company's human resources department, and friends who know the best doctors. They get the best care available. In fact, overtreatment is a bigger problem for this group than undertreatment. Their chief complaint with the health care system is that health care costs are too high, but mostly they aren't avoiding care because they can't pay for it. They are sometimes shocked at the cost of their prescriptions, but they can usually afford them. While a single major medical event like cancer can result in significant financial challenges, they don't live in constant fear of bankruptcy.

The other half of the country faces a different set of health care challenges. They often work low-paying jobs, sometimes more than one at time. They don't have much in the way of savings. English may not be their first language. They may live in a small town without much access to health care providers, or in a city with few affordable health care practitioners. Many in this group use the emergency room when they need health care, often postponing it until they are very sick. They may be uninsured, or on Medicare or Medicaid, or on a subsidized Obamacare insurance plan. Even if they are insured, any unplanned medical expense could easily bankrupt them. Forty percent of Americans who receive a cancer diagnosis spend their entire life savings within two years.[2] While the Peloton crowd has a Whole Foods near their house, this group is more likely to have a convenience store like a 7-Eleven or a fast-food restaurant. If they have access to fresh food, it is harder to afford. Being poor means facing a variety of obstacles: there's less access to nutritious food, affordable and safe housing is often out of reach, reliable transportation may be a problem, child care is too expensive. And then there's the problem of managing the inherent trauma associated with poverty. All of this makes getting health care and staying healthy more difficult. In my speeches, I refer to this group as the "take-the-bus crowd."

Since the early 1980s, the disparity in how people live in America has grown larger and larger. In 1983, upper-income families had 28 times the wealth of lower-income families. In 2016, they had 75 times the wealth. This shows up in the outcomes people get from the health care system. Where you live, zip code by zip code, is a good approximation for your income and race, and a difference of a few miles can mean a difference of as much as 30 years of life expectancy within the same city.

Even if you eliminate income, race-based disparities are daunting. Black women are three to four times more likely to die in childbirth than white women. Race-based disparities are likewise stark for cancer, heart disease, mental illness, and almost any other health problem you can think of.[3]

During COVID-19, these disparities dramatically affected who lived and who died. Working people who had very little savings and would have no income if they missed work, like Ahmed, were more likely to be exposed to the virus, and suffered disproportionately. Because the people who were required to work and interact with the public were the same people who lacked access to affordable medical care, the United States was set up for negative health care outcomes that would disproportionately hit communities that historically have been left behind. Black, indigenous, and people of color communities would be especially hard hit, with their jobs, their living conditions, their access to care, and embedded racism combining for a deadly mix.

Unequal access to health and health care services felt like a buried land mine for all but the most-well-off Americans. And as with all land mines, even if you could avoid them for a while, God help you when you couldn't. There were other barely hidden land mines when COVID-19 struck. The chronic underinvestment in public health that our Cassandras had pointed out and a country growing openly hostile to institutions and experts. The Trump administration had weakened precisely the professional agencies we would need to rely on when something went wrong. Only the slightest additional pressure would trigger a massive explosion.

The Stepchildren of Health Care

In December 2019, I was asked to give the keynote speech at the 50th-anniversary celebration for the University of Minnesota's School of Public Health.[4] Before I prepared that speech, I hadn't given much thought to the role public health played in our lives.

One definition of public health I've seen is the prevention of disease and the prolonging of life. As important as it sounds, public health professionals are in a sense the odd ducks of the U.S. health care system. Unlike other roles in health care, public health jobs are not high-paying and normally aren't very visible. And the government and pharmaceutical companies do not line up to give research money to public health, unlike other fields of health care. To me, the goal of public health is to make the world safer for us and future generations. The crises public health professionals address are not the acute ones individuals run to the emergency room with but the large ones that are everywhere but largely invisible and so are easier to ignore. Congress has felt little urgency to invest in their work.

In fact, public health in America has been a huge success. Americans at the end of the twentieth century were living 30 years longer than at the century's start.[5] While public health doesn't get all the credit for this, it has had a massive impact across the United States and the globe. Those who worked in public health could rattle off the series of initiatives that have extended life across the globe: Clean water and air. The reduction in smoking. Defeating smallpox and polio and eventually winning the day on AIDS. Public health professionals will also point to all the horrors we didn't experience that we'll never know about thanks to these advances. Most of what they've accomplished is taken for granted by society.

For all of its success, public health has been seeing less and less investment in this country. Since the 2008 recession, local public health departments, once the beacons of a healthier country, have lost 55,000 workers, a quarter of their workforce. The United States now spends just 2.5 percent of its health care budget on public health and prevention, 30 percent less than a decade ago. The other 97.5 percent goes largely to the costs of illness. We spend a meager $274 per person on public health. For that investment, public health is supposed to address a litany of challenges, including the opioid addiction crisis, climbing obesity rates, contaminated water, the suicide crisis—and pandemic prevention.[6]

Other countries, including some of the poorest nations in the world, have far better public health infrastructures. As *The Atlantic* science writer Ed Yong pointed out, in the war-torn Democratic Republic of Congo (DRC), local health workers and the WHO traced two and a half times as many contacts per day of those infected during that country's 2019 Ebola outbreak as Maryland has done during COVID-19. The difference is that the DRC had a contact tracing infrastructure in place, whereas Maryland had to hire and train workers from scratch. The United States has been a victim of its own success—because we have not faced the public health crises that the DRC has, we've become complacent and investment has been diminished. The CDC's budget for public health has been cut by 10 percent in the last decade, and President Trump has repeatedly proposed further cuts to the CDC.[7]

An important part of our public health infrastructure is the Strategic National Stockpile (SNS). This is a repository of drugs, vaccines, and medical supplies that Congress first authorized in 1999, to replenish and supplement state and local supplies during emergencies. It is overseen by the Department of Health and Human Services, in coordination with the Department of Homeland Security. In 2009, responding to the swine flu epidemic, the SNS distributed 85 million N95 masks. Since then, the masks have not been replenished. In 2011, President Obama asked Congress for $650 million to replenish the stockpile but was denied by the Republican House; instead, they introduced a bill the following year to cut stockpile funding by 10 percent. During the Zika and Ebola outbreaks, Obama requested additional funding for the stockpile, but Congress cut those requests in half. During the Trump years, those requests were discontinued. In March, at the beginning of the coronavirus outbreak, the stockpile contained only about 12 million of the 3.5 billion N95 masks that federal officials estimated the health care system would need to fight this pandemic. Complacency played a role, but so did ideology. Anti-government GOP rhetoric and tax cuts for the wealthy and corporations were a clear priority.[8]

The night of my speech to 1,000 people in the McNamara Center in downtown Minneapolis, COVID-19 had just begun to spread undetected in Wuhan, China. My speech was a battle cry for public health to stop toiling in the dark and start competing for massive investment dollars. To some audible gasps, I proposed the creation of a plan to get $100 billion from Congress and take public health out from the shadows. Given the events of that night on the other side of the world, that suggestion turned out to be on the mark, but way too late in coming. Soon we were spending trillions of dollars catching up to a problem we hadn't taken steps to prevent.

From Obama to Trump

On January 19, 2017, I stood in front of my office at Health and Human Services in Washington, D.C., and watched as the framed photographs of Barack Obama and Joe Biden were taken down from the wall. The following day, I knew, they would be replaced with those of Donald Trump and Mike Pence. The next day, January 20, while a crowd of Trump's supporters gathered on the Mall to watch the new president get sworn in, I drove to Andrews Air Force Base to watch the outgoing president and first lady board Air Force One and fly out of the capital one final time. They took pictures with people who were there to wish them well, and I caught up with a number of friends I had made in the time I was in the administration. It wasn't until the plane took off and I was driving back to my nearly empty apartment that I thought about what was ahead for the country.

As one of the people shutting things down at the end of the Obama administration, I had several important priorities. We "ran through the tape," as my boss, HHS secretary Sylvia Burwell, liked to say, serving people up to the last minute and getting a few things done that we anticipated would be neglected in the new administration.

Whichever agency you look at, whether it's the CMS, FDA, CDC, or FBI, there are thousands of people—career civil servants—who do vital work that keeps the country running. As new administrations come in, of either party, the civil servants maintain their focus on the public they serve even as they welcome their new bosses. Most new administrations come in with the humility to appreciate the institutional knowledge that exists only in career civil servants, and time spent serving with them only serves to grow the respect for that expertise.

One of the most important duties in a democracy is to orchestrate a smooth transition between one administration and the next. Around the government, each of us prepared extensive memos for the Trump team in which we captured everything we knew and everything we had learned. Ninety percent of the operations of government are about making the processes work and not getting trapped in easily preventable mistakes. Generations of learned rules, customs, and idiosyncrasies are maintained and documented so that each succeeding administration benefits from the ones before it.

At the start of 2017 there was one problem: the Trump administration wasn't interested in protocol and lessons learned. Trump, who characterized the career workforce as, variously, the "deep state" or the "swamp," thought of civil servants as his own employees, introducing loyalty oaths and nondisclosure agreements and making it clear dissent was not welcome. Trump and his team were also confident they possessed all the knowledge they needed. All across the federal government, from the White House to the agencies, these memos went unread. In HHS, they didn't want to know how Obama's people had done things. My successor at the CMS, Seema Verma, actually did meet with me off-site twice, but she was the exception. The incoming HHS secretary, Tom Price, refused to meet with Secretary Burwell. This was the norm.

Of course, one of the most crucial elements of the 2016 transition plan was preparation for a global pandemic. There is no "commonsense" or "instinctual" way to respond to a pandemic. There are right moves that must be made in the right order, quickly, and with limited information. A viral outbreak at some point in the future was a near certainty, and it would likely start overseas, probably in the Middle East, Africa, or Asia, where most of the recent outbreaks had begun. The most important step was quick containment before it spread in the community and became too difficult to track. Once that happened, it would be like trying to contain an invisible wildfire.

When the Ebola outbreak occurred in October 2014, President Obama hired Ron Klain to oversee the federal response. Ron was a lawyer and senior Democratic advisor who had represented Al Gore in the 2000 election recount in Florida. In 2021, he would become Joe Biden's chief of staff, to many the most powerful job in Washington. As a senior advisor for Biden's pandemic response, he was the ideal boss. At the outset of Ebola, what Klain lacked in public health background, he more than made up for in operational focus, his well-earned respect from peers, knowledge of government, and his calm, decisive demeanor.

Having contained Ebola, Ron and the team assembled the collective operational knowledge about pandemics that had been acquired and created the Playbook for High-Consequence Emerging Infectious Disease Threats and Biological Incidents, aka "the Playbook."[9] A 69-page manual for all future administrations, the Playbook contained detailed instructions for a coordinated response from departments and agencies including HHS, Defense, Homeland Security, State, Labor, Transportation, Agriculture, Environmental Protection, and the intelligence community. Without clear assignment of responsibilities, a quick response from all those agencies would be nearly impossible, costing valuable time and lives.

President Obama also set up an apparatus called the Directorate for Global Health Security and Biodefense to make sure prevention and containment could happen without delay. This was important.[10] Any delays getting started meant the difference between small campfires and raging wildfires.

Trump eliminated the directorate and tossed out the Playbook.[11] If the White House were on fire and all the fire trucks said "Obama" on them, Trump surely would have let it burn to the ground.

Trump, Inc. Takes on the Deep State

Many Trump appointees had utter contempt for the mission of their agencies and a deep hostility to government regulation. Particularly where consumer protections or government services of any kind were concerned, Trump's aim was to undermine his own agencies. The Consumer Financial Protection Bureau, created to protect consumers against predatory lenders, was put under the control of its leading opponent, Mick Mulvaney, who slowly dismantled it and brought the agency's work to a near halt. The Environmental Protection Agency was similarly put under the control of its leading critic, Scott Pruitt. Under Trump, the EPA rolled back automobile fuel efficiency standards, loosened controls on toxic ash from coal plants, and relaxed restrictions on mercury emissions.[12]

I had several memorable encounters with Trump cabinet members. Ben Carson, secretary of Housing and Urban Development, was a frequent diner in many of the best restaurants in Washington. On my trips into D.C., I would see him having a $100 breakfast at the Hay-Adams Hotel, or out to dinner with friends. One evening a few months after the inauguration, I was meeting then-Congressman Joe Kennedy for dinner in a Capitol Hill restaurant. Natalie Davis, my senior advisor, was with me, and we had a drink while waiting for Joe and one of his staff members.

Carson was sitting in the booth closest to us with his wife and another couple. Whenever the noise died down, we could overhear Carson disparaging the people he served and the staff at HUD.

"The deep state is real," he said.

"Why can't you just wipe them out?" one of his guests asked.

Career civil service protections were in place for precisely these reasons.

(Later on we overheard another gem. "The homeless people think they own the park," the man in charge of housing the poor said. I still mull that over.)

This attitude prevailed through the pre-pandemic Trump administration: FBI and State Department civil servants would be tweeted about derisively, whistleblowers would be exposed, important regulations overturned. It was more than just business for Trump. It was a common refrain among his large donors: "We've allowed these unelected bureaucrats who hate corporations to make all the rules."

In truth, career civil servants are an incredible national asset—
not to mention as dedicated a group as you will find. They may work
for decades to become experts in a sometimes narrow but important field. There are civil servants whose entire career may be spent
understanding what happens if Pakistan attacks India—something
that's not very useful up until the moment Pakistan attacks India,
when it becomes priceless. Occasionally a federal employee will be
tempted by a higher salary and move to a private-sector company.
Frequently, they come back after a short time. The explanation is
always the same: they miss the purpose and the mission of serving
the public. Having managed large private and public-sector work-
forces, I wouldn't trade the CMS team for anyone.

Scientific agencies such as the Centers for Disease Control were a
particular target for Trump. Like the strategic stockpile, the CDC was
a perfect place to cut—invisible, out of sight of the public, something
the president didn't understand, was unlikely to notice, and didn't
think he'd need. The CDC is our principal public health agency, with
premier scientists working across the globe. Trump diminished it financially and hurt its capabilities in ways that were felt when the pandemic began. Funding cuts forced the agency to reduce or discontinue
epidemic-prevention efforts in 39 out of 49 countries. These operations were what allowed us to gather valuable intelligence. When a
highly contagious disease broke out and time made all the difference,
that capability gave the United States the opportunity to get ahead of
it. Among the countries where efforts were scaled back was China.
In the 2020 budget, Trump proposed a 10 percent budget cut for the
CDC, amounting to about $750 million—peanuts compared to the
trillions of dollars in COVID-19 relief that Congress would soon request once the pandemic began to overwhelm the country.[13]

Something else changed about the CDC during the Trump presidency. When Tom Frieden directed the agency under the Obama
administration, he kept a quote on the wall in his office:

Promoting science isn't just about providing resources—it is
also about protecting free and open inquiry. It is about letting

scientists . . . do their jobs, free from manipulation or coercion, and listening to what they tell us, even when it's inconvenient—especially when it's inconvenient. It is about ensuring that scientific data is never distorted or concealed to serve a political agenda—and that we make scientific decisions based on facts, not ideology.[14]

The quote was from Barack Obama.

Not only were resources not being provided under the Trump administration to prepare for a pandemic, but Trump's philosophy was 180 degrees away from Obama's. Trump did not tolerate any opinion that differed from his own. He reshaped the CDC by adding five political appointees inside the agency, where there had never been more than one.[15] During the pandemic, he and HHS secretary Alex Azar installed Michael Caputo, a communications specialist at HHS, to review and approve the CDC's work and its external communications.

The man Trump put in charge of the CDC, Robert Redfield, is most often described to me as "a nice guy." What typically follows that description is the assessment that he lacked the expertise to run the agency even in normal times, and was way over his head throughout the COVID-19 crisis. What Redfield was best known for before heading the CDC was his opposition to condom use in the early years of the AIDS epidemic. An evangelical Christian, he was part of a group that pushed abstinence education to control the spread of AIDS.[16]

Nods to the evangelical base were a big factor in Trump's appointment process. Once in government, Trump clearly prized loyalists who wouldn't question him, wouldn't overreach, and wouldn't align themselves with the career staff, whom he distrusted. But whether his appointees were weak or loyal, the effect was the same.

The staff CDC scientists, those who remained, were some of the best in the world. But as Tom Frieden told me, they were deeply demoralized. Larry Brilliant, the preeminent expert in pandemics, was even blunter when we talked about it in July 2020:

My beloved CDC, which for all of us who fancy ourselves epidemiologists, CDC is a little bit like Mecca. We've all gone there
at one time or another believing that that was the center of such
integrity and great science. And still has phenomenal scientists
and great integrity. It is either forgotten or it is being suppressed,
and I believe it's being suppressed.[17]

The Pandemic Meets the Cultural Divide

Donald Trump's supporters found in him something more than
just a president or policy agenda. Trump gave them permission to
be who they wanted to be, even if that meant offending others.
Those who expected civility and decency out of the president,
and those who were slighted by Trump—often women, the poor,
people of color, immigrants, people with preexisting illnesses—
were outraged not just by Trump but by his supporters.

Taming a virus is a simple matter of reducing its circulation.
When not wearing a mask became a cultural or political statement
during the COVID-19 outbreak, it created an unexpected twist. Surveys showed 70 percent of Democrats saying they wear a mask "every time" compared to 37 percent of Republicans.[18] The scientist Bill
Joy put together an analysis showing that for each 10 percent of the
population that goes about everyday life with minimal precautions,
100,000 more people are expected to die. So even small cracks can
become huge ruptures, and the virus becomes harder to control. The
wealthiest countries in the world turned out not to be the best at
fighting COVID-19. The countries that have more social cohesion
have all the advantage.

▪▪▪

Before the pandemic even started, America had been flirting with
disaster for years. The dangers of an unequal society and health
care system exposed many to higher risks; the diminishment of

public health, of civil servants, and of our important institutions left us flat-footed when it came time to respond to new dangers; and our increased polarization created an environment where a small failure to manage the pandemic could turn into a large one. And, unfortunately, our failures were hardly small.

CHAPTER 3

WAKING UP LATE

Scene: Your Town, U.S.A.

On the morning of February 25, 2020, Dr. Nancy Messonnier, the director of the National Center for Immunization and Respiratory Diseases at the CDC, spoke to the press about the looming threat of COVID-19. "It's not a question of if this [coronavirus pandemic] will happen but when this will happen and how many people in this country will have severe illnesses." She went on to say, "Disruptions to everyday life may be severe, but people might want to start thinking about that now."[1] She hinted at some dramatic-sounding things: school closures, businesses moving meetings online, hospitals postponing elective surgeries, and avoiding large gatherings. She was remarkably prescient.

But Messonnier's key attribute wasn't her prescience I realized after getting to know her. It was her honesty. She broke ranks, and her comment was followed by a drop in the stock market.

The president's response to a woman with a distinguished and proud record of service to the public and science? He threatened to fire her.[2] Health and Human Services Secretary Alex Azar went about destroying her reputation for not being a team player.

Larry Kudlow, the head of the National Economic Council, almost immediately went on television to reassure the nation: "We have contained this. I won't say airtight, but pretty close to airtight."[3] Azar falsely described the virus as "contained" the same day.[4]

Less than two years after President Trump disbanded the National Security Council's Directorate for Global Health Security and Biodefense, a pandemic hit the United States. Trump and his political advisors would consistently eschew the advice of public health experts.[5] Trump claimed that the media's focus on the pandemic was designed to make him look bad and distract from his reelection story.[6] As we now know, despite his public comments, Trump admitted to journalist Bob Woodward that he was aware as early as February that COVID-19 was deadly, highly infectious, and coming to the United States.[7]

Shortly after the Messonnier event, Mike Pence's press secretary, Katie Miller, issued a directive that HHS was not permitted to issue any communication that raised concern among the public. Secretary Azar proposed talking points that said things were under control but "could change rapidly." Miller soundly rejected that statement and pulled Azar from a planned appearance on *Fox & Friends* the next morning. He was prohibited from doing any media for 45 days.

Each day Trump didn't act counted. Remember Zach's math: we weren't facing spread from 1 to 2 to 3 to 4 to 5, but from 1 to 2 to 4 to 8 to 16. Each day we didn't acknowledge the bug meant a day lost in terms of acquiring the needed testing supplies and masks, for which the global supply was limited. Each day we still didn't have the ability to test was a day we couldn't locate outbreaks. And, most important, when something is spreading invisibly and exponentially, each day we didn't inform the public was a day the virus became harder to control.

Despite Trump's disappointing and harmful response, I had no interest in going after the president publicly at that point. Rather, I saw the virus itself as the enemy. This view was informed by math, not politics. The virus needed humans to circulate. Our freedom-loving democracy would have a difficult time taking universally strong measures the way China had. The best we could hope for was to keep politics away from our pandemic response. If only half the country complied with public health guidelines, the virus would not go away until there were good vaccines available. That was the math. At some point, I was sure, Trump would have no choice but to acknowledge the pandemic, and once he did, I hoped he would remain engaged as long as possible.

In most other countries, the pandemic response had little to do with which political party was in control. In the United States, there was very little that wasn't political. Many Democrats don't know a single Republican, and vice versa. As Michael Burgess, a conservative congressman from Texas, once told me, "Not only is Democrat a bad word in my district, but so is bipartisanship. If you ever see me in public, please just look the other way." (If I wrote here that Burgess was a nice guy who once drove me to the Capitol for a hearing I was late for, he would probably be booed out of town and replaced with someone more conservative.)

And so I put this out on my Twitter feed:

> A message to the people who turn to this account for health care politics, which includes sharp & well-earned criticism of Trump & his policies. In the face of Coronavirus, I am turning my attention to where I think it is most needed—to help us all defeat this together. The White House, HHS, state governors of either party, members of Congress know how to reach me & can't be afraid to keep doing it. We're on the same side here.
>
> I'm told the virus spreads from Trump supporter to Biden supporter to Bernie supporter and back. There are too many problems—and indeed solutions—to fight each other. More masks, ventilators, [diagnostic] tests, more ICUs, [there is] anxiety we all feel. Everybody: DoD, VA, FEMA, National Guard, Army Corps of Engineers, elected lawmakers & critics need to pull together.[8]

We had to strive for more cohesion or we would pay for it in loss of life. When I got asked about the president on TV, which was practically every day, I would answer by saying, "We have to navigate from where we are, not from where we wish we were," and then talk about what I believed we needed to get done to save lives.

MSNBC host Kasie Hunt asked me to compare and contrast the polar opposite recommendations from two congresspeople, Alexandria Ocasio-Cortez (AOC) and Devin Nunes. There may not be two members of Congress who were a stronger litmus test of your politics. AOC favored Medicare for All and the Green New Deal. Republicans had made her their new boogeyman. Nunes was the man Democrats hated because they believed he had buried the Trump campaign's collusion with Russian interference during the 2016 election. AOC asked people to stay in and not dine out at bars and restaurants, while Nunes echoed the White House line that the virus was a hoax and encouraged people to eat out.[9]

Hunt wanted to know whose advice people should follow.

"This isn't about Democrats or Republicans," I replied. "Find your own trusted sources, people in your city or in your state. We've been chasing this problem instead of getting ahead of it. It's in New York in a big way, but if I was in a city with no community spread, I might take Congressman Nunes's advice. But as soon as you live in a city with community spread, whether they close the bars and restaurants or not, stay home. It's a short period in your life." I consider Nunes one of the most unimpressive people in Washington, and saying something neutral about him took impressive restraint.

The Governors

John Doerr was right to challenge me to make my concerns known publicly. Hundreds of thousands of people were following my tweets on the pandemic to understand what was happening. But sparking real action in the country with the president working so hard against it would take some work—more than "Twitter work," as Lana would say. One of my mantras when I was facing daily crises during the ACA turnaround, where every minute counted, involved how to deal with things that aren't going your way. If someone came to me with a problem they couldn't solve and they were just spinning, I would always say the same thing: "When things aren't happening the way you want, just focus on what you can control today and don't worry about the rest." That described where we were in early March 2020. So I decided to try my luck with our nation's governors, mayors, and state health secretaries and health commissioners.

The federal government has specialized resources built for a pandemic response, including large disaster recovery agencies, large numbers of military and civilian personnel, nationwide stockpiles, special contracting authority, the power of the purse, the authority to increase production of essential goods, and the ability to coordinate a response across multiple states. States, on the other hand, were less than an ideal place to center responsibility for the response to COVID-19. Governors' budgets and disaster response resources weren't anything close to sufficient. The last thing we needed was to have 50-plus approaches and 50-plus bidders for goods and services in short supply. But in the face of likely mass casualties and a weak federal response, governors were the next-best option. They controlled public communication channels, had public health resources, and had authority to declare emergencies. If Trump didn't act, governors would end up owning the crisis.

No governor ran for office expecting a global pandemic, and each governor I spoke with was in a different state of awareness about it. None had the needed infrastructure—and why would they? Juliette Kayyem, a former Homeland Security official in the Obama administration, explained to me that, in general, we typically prepared for two types of disasters: national disasters, handled by the federal government, and more localized disasters, handled by state governments with help from FEMA or the National Guard.[10] Because the president was largely sitting on his hands, this was turning into a new thing—a 50-state disaster without overarching federal support.

On March 7, I put together a brief memo for about a dozen

governors designed to help them accelerate a start-up response. I got quick input from the best people who could help state leaders anticipate what was to come. In addition to Mike Osterholm, I called on Rob Califf, the former head of the FDA, who gave me an estimate of when scientific progress on therapies and vaccines would be made. Sun Microsystems founder Bill Joy, who had been studying pandemics for more than a decade, shared with me the lessons learned from the Wuhan outbreak. Kevin Conroy, CEO of diagnostic lab Exact Sciences, helped me estimate when diagnostic tests might be available in sufficient supply around the country—he thought it would be at least six weeks. Rod Hochman, the CEO of Providence St. Joseph Health, the largest hospital system in Washington State, gave me the rundown on what had been learned from the early outbreak in Seattle. Ron Klain, who had run the Ebola task force under President Obama, helped me pin down the things leaders should prioritize. Tom Frieden, former head of the CDC, who had also run New York City's famed Department of Health, told me how a governor could differentiate a good public health advisor from a bad one—an important task, since many governors would need to find them quickly. People who had on-the-ground experience with the CDC's Epidemic Intelligence Service were of particular value.

What I ended up sending was a three-page memo starting with the most important things they needed to do.

1. *Prevention now will be easier than clean-up later. Controlling 10 people is easier than 100, 1000, 10,000, 100,000. That's how it vectors. Act while your job is easier. You are not overdoing it.*
2. *The number one public interest and concern is safety. State government needs to showcase transparency, competence, and credibility.*
3. *It's already in your state and many of your communities and you should make plans to act assuming you are both the front line and last line. Federal money, kits, and eventually a*

vaccine and treatments will show up at some point, but move forward assuming little Federal support.

4. *Experts believe we are already past the person-to-person stage of transmission and in community transmission in most large communities.*

5. *Infection controls and protocols are poor in health care settings to begin with. Assume there are sufficient deficiencies that need to be closed.*

6. *You can't do everything. Start with the highest risk areas (nursing homes, hospitals, travelers) and go from there. Allocate resources—dollars and people. To emphasize, long-term care and elder facilities are at enormous risk.*

7. *Let public health officials guide your decisions and provide them the support they need. Protect them from excessive meetings and PR requests.*

8. *An important principle is that the weakest link in the community will drive infection development. International travel, major metropolitan area commuters, elderly populations. Incubation periods and spreading methods make it hard for people to self-identify.*

9. *The numbers of infected will grow dramatically in the next weeks as testing increases. Make sure the public sees this is not an increase in spread but a baselining and no reason to panic.*

10. *A tight chain of command is critical. Staffing, resources, scorecard development, communication protocols, and budget are important early actions.*

11. *The situation will be very fluid. These are phase 1 basic recommendations. If the virus begins to spread rapidly, protocols will need to change.*

As far as I was concerned, the ability to follow these 11 points would separate those governors who were successful from those who weren't. The next two pages of the memo were a playbook on launching emergency operations from a standing start: they elaborated on hiring, structuring a SWAT team, personnel, messaging, and daily reporting. I had stood up state command centers in a matter of a week and felt like it was one thing I could do in my sleep.

I sent the memo out, and questions and requests for help immediately came in from a dozen states. Two minutes after I texted the memo to her, Governor Kate Brown of Oregon wrote back and asked for help. Annie Lamont, the first lady in Connecticut, asked how to handle three people diagnosed with COVID-19 who had been at a basketball game and a Starbucks; she asked me to get on the phone with the governor and talk about protocols. Colorado governor Jared Polis and I walked through the memo together, and he texted to find out where to get PPE, and later to help find ventilators, and later still to ask about nursing home safety.

Governors and their staffs were feeling the immense burden of the lack of a national response to the crisis. Many were already stretched thin just managing day-to-day government functions. With help from the team at United States of Care, we created a rapid-response effort to help with incoming needs and to share best practices among states on a regular basis. We also put this information online for everyone to see. In Michigan, even my sister, Lesley, jumped in. With no background in either health care or logistics, she was soon managing the stand-up of a Detroit field hospital and point-of-care testing in the state.

There was another call I needed to make—to my Town Hall Ventures partners Trevor Price and David Whelan. They were both living in New York City and had been hearing rumors that the city might shut down.

David, an Australian with years of experience operating in complex and strategic environments, had an outsider's view of the U.S. health care system. Australians, like Americans, value independence and individualism, but he could never understand why our country's health care system left so many people to fend for themselves. He didn't hesitate in his response: "Mate, go work on the country's problems. It's a national emergency. I've got your back."

"I've got your back" may be the most welcome four words in

the English language. His response reminded me of the day when I told Lana I had been asked to go to Washington to try to turn around the failing ACA exchanges in 2013. Almost immediately she said, "Good. Don't come home until it's fixed."

Trevor was a mix of skeptical New Englander and visionary. He was feeling the heavy burden of what could happen to underserved communities in New York. I told him to look out for his family, but he didn't want to talk about that. "I've got to do something to help the most vulnerable New Yorkers," he said. "We can't just watch this crisis happen."

Within weeks, Trevor had enlisted 85 companies to his cause, including some of the largest technology and health care companies in the country. They donated telemedicine services, free transportation, grocery delivery, and other things that would help keep those New Yorkers who were at highest risk free from infection. Soon, older and low-income people around the city started getting text messages every morning that read: "How are you? Need anything?" Everything from grocery delivery to mental health services was offered at no cost. United States of Care documented the process and created a playbook on how this was done, for use in other states. Wouldn't it be nice if health care always worked so simply?

How Bad Could It Be?

How many lives could we lose in this pandemic? This was a question I tried hard to avoid discussing, particularly in those early days. First of all, it depended on so many things. How soon would there be a vaccine? How well would it work? Would we find therapies that worked? But mostly, in the early days, it depended on how quickly the virus circulated. And that depended on how much we would change the way we behaved and how long that could be sustained. I was suspicious of anyone who believed this could be easily predicted.

In the early stages, scientists were attempting to answer a different question: How many people would die in the United States if we did nothing? This was relevant because at the time we were doing nothing. A group of scientists in California concluded that the deaths would be in the millions. Mike Osterholm estimated it could be about 800,000.[11] Imperial College London released a paper that became highly visible, estimating the number of deaths at over 2 million. Tom Frieden estimated a worst-case but not impossible scenario of 1 million deaths.[12] Matthew Biggerstaff, a scientist at the CDC, estimated a midpoint of 950,000 deaths and a worst case of 1.7 million people. But I was sure we would never reach those worst-case numbers: even if the government did nothing, we citizens would react, because that's what humans do. So these felt less like predictions than theoretical estimates. Anthony Fauci, speaking in front of Congress on March 11, said, "I can't give you a realistic number until we put into the factor of how we respond. If we're complacent and don't do really aggressive containment and mitigation, the number could go way up and be involved in many, many millions."

In many ways, all these numbers served to numb people as much as shock them. What's 1,000 more people when the numbers are so large?

As the death toll climbed in March, Trump began to use the worst-case numbers to make the claim that his actions—primarily banning travel from China—saved many lives: in late March it was "tens of thousands"; by early April it was "hundreds of thousands";[13] in July that number was millions.[14] Of course, Trump didn't actually ban all travel from China. As mentioned in the introduction, nearly 40,000 people traveled to the United States from China without quarantine in the months after the supposed travel ban.[15] And much of the worst of the virus came to the United States not from China but from Europe.[16] Some parts of the world that maintained travel with China, such as Hong Kong, did far better than the United States. In truth, Trump didn't do much of anything to reduce the spread.

I preferred to talk about the projected death toll in a different way: individually. Drawing on Zach's simple analysis, I reiterated over and over that each of us had the ability to save 40 lives by our actions. People needed to imagine faces, not columns of numbers. But on one occasion, I put forward the bigger-picture view. On March 12, so that the public could see what the experts were saying, I wrote on Twitter, "Currently experts expect over 1 million deaths in the U.S. since the virus was not contained & we cannot even test for it. This will be recorded as a major preventable public health disaster."[17] I added that the number of people who died was very much under our control and not our destiny.

A few weeks later, tweets began to appear from Trump supporters who felt that bad news about the virus amounted to criticism of the president: "Slavitt's the guy who predicted a million people would die!" I hadn't, of course, but I felt certain that those who had made such terrifying predictions had a strong basis for saying so. I was hit with the accusation commonly thrown at everyone in public health: that I was fearmongering.

In early March, John Doerr and I spoke almost every evening. He was even more worried than I was. More than a decade earlier, he'd been persuaded by a group of engineers and thinkers including Bill Gates, Bill Joy, and Larry Brilliant that a pandemic on the order of the influenza in 1918 was coming. So in 2006 he had started a fund to invest in pandemic prevention and management. It was John who introduced me to Bill Joy.

At first blush, Bill Joy couldn't have had a name less suited to his temperament. He had publicly predicted a pandemic like COVID-19 in a 2008 TED Talk, nearly a decade before other big names in science.[18] Since the outbreak began in Wuhan, he had been hunkered down in his Florida home. The doom and gloom he shared were hard to take at times. But there was almost nobody I learned more from than Bill about what to expect as the pandemic unfolded. His knowledge of the intricate details of how rapidly the virus could spread and how little we were doing to mitigate that led to a deep pessimism. He understood the damage a pathogen like this could cause, and his anger and bitter disappointment that the country was not ready showed.

Some gems he shared with me included the fact that COVID-19 can remain in people's respiratory tract for up to 37 days, more than twice as long as the recommended isolation period; that the recommended six feet of social distance had no basis in science; that death rates in the United States would be much higher than in other countries because of our higher rates of obesity and chronic illness (he believed 41 percent of adults could be at risk because of such co-morbidities); that even if people isolated at home, family spread would be lethal; and that day care centers would end up driving infections in our medical personnel. Most frighteningly, drawing on the work of evolutionary biologist Paul Ewald, he believed that a virus like COVID-19, especially because it could be spread by asymptomatic carriers, could evolve to be more lethal while it was spreading, turning into "a monster threat."

And those were the cheerful conversations.

In too many cases, his early concerns, at one point apocryphal, would prove accurate. For every hour I spent on the phone with Bill I got the equivalent of a PhD's worth of knowledge. He read every study, knew every bit of evidence, could do exponential math in his head, and was modeling the virus's impact out months ahead of where we were. I once asked Bill how trust in a vaccine would impact the duration and deadliness of the pandemic. Instead of answering directly, he built me an entire model in about an hour so I could alter the variables myself. What struck me later, upon reflection, was that everything I learned from Bill was knowledge available to the Trump administration. What at one point felt like sleeping through the alarm I began to understand as the Trump administration choosing to turn the alarm off to keep us asleep.

Bill believed there was only one valid solution: forced isolation of anyone infected. He argued that early evidence out of Wuhan and a Harvard biostatistics study showed that, short of a vaccine, the only way to defeat the virus was for a centralized government to mandate separation and quarantining of everyone infected, and then to trace every contact of each infected person and force those contacts to isolate, even if that meant separating family members.

Bill's approach would have crushed the virus in short order, much as we saw happen in China. Purely on the science he may have been dead right, but there was no need to tell Bill that Americans would never stand for kids being separated from their parents. (Okay, white kids would never be separated from their parents.) He knew it, and it frustrated him to no end that we didn't have the stomach to kill the bug.

John, Bill, and I decided that in the face of inaction and out-and-out misinformation from the government, we needed to take on the daunting task of persuading the public to stay indoors and hide from an invisible enemy—an enemy that, if they succeeded in evading it, they might believe never existed at all. That enemy lingered in the air, in the laughter and tears and voices of their friends and loved ones, in close quarters, and in large crowds.

That challenge embodies the key conundrum of fighting any pandemic: the more successful you are in preventing its spread, the harder it gets to convince people that past and future interventions were and will be necessary.

I thought about what it must be like at the CDC at this moment. Many people who knew what was going on felt silenced after Nancy Messonnier was nearly fired for speaking up. At this point, I assumed they were no longer able to get a consistent message out to the public. The public messaging from the White House was that the virus was temporary and flu-like, and that masks were not needed.

We had to change the message.

#StayHome

Asking people to voluntarily isolate and take other safety measures was obviously a far cry from Bill Joy's call for the government to mandate such behavior. Getting any meaningful level of compliance was a long shot, but it was the only play we had. Politics and culture in the United States were unlike those in the rest of the world. The Chinese government took severe and bold measures, including isolating anyone positive for COVID-19 in quarantine dormitories, and in weeks they had smashed the virus in Wuhan, saving a lot of lives in the process.[19] Other countries pulled together to bring the case count down to near zero. Each country had its own emphasis, demonstrating how basic public health practices could be adapted culture by culture. The Czech Republic was one of the first to implement universal mask wearing.[20] Greece instituted a strict system of penalties for ignoring social distancing guidelines.[21] Japan and Singapore put the collective good ahead of individual self-interest and enforced public health guidelines such as mandatory masking and closing places where the spread was most common. New Zealand used a system of color coding to communicate to the public when and where the virus had spread and greater precautions must be taken.[22] In Germany, Chancellor Angela Merkel's news conferences were a master class in science, providing ongoing education on the virus and on the necessity of public health policies.[23] Within a month of Germany's first case, contact tracing was implemented nationwide and large gatherings and travel were restricted.[24]

In comparison to most of these other countries, the American public was impatient, untrusting, and unaccustomed to sacrificing individual rights for the public good. The political and legal system made enforcing broad federal public health measures tricky; such efforts relied mostly on a 75-year-old law, the Public Health Service Act, and a two-century-old legal precedent, *Gibbons v. Ogden*. Despite the obvious looming threat, no one with authority or credibility was calling on the American people to change their behaviors to protect themselves and others.

Communicating clearly in a way that resonated with the public, provided practical recommendations, and included fact-based explanations would be essential. Saying, "A microscopic virus is coming. You won't see it but it might kill you or people you love" probably wasn't a good idea. Nor did I like "Flatten the curve," as it made the pandemic sound like it would be over after a short-lived effort to spread things out—which was highly unlikely. The phrase "social distance" implied a kind of isolation we did not need; in fact, maintaining social connections would be more important than ever. What we needed was a short, direct, and straightforward phrase that also evoked a level of action.

On March 12, I laid out for John a public campaign to convince everyone who was able to physically isolate to do so voluntarily. We decided to make the focus of the campaign #StayHome (sometimes seen as #StayHomeSaveLives—and occasionally as #StaytheFHome).

As I sat down to map out a manifesto for this unprecedented effort, I tried to put myself at the kitchen tables of the people whose lives were being disrupted by the arrival of this unexpected and little-understood public health emergency: people who worked in offices, shops, and restaurants, factory and warehouse workers, students and teachers, health care providers, public safety officers, bus drivers and airline employees, and countless others not sure what was happening or how to respond. Many Americans were scared but lacked clear information about how to stay safe; others were frozen with indecision about which precautions to take or whether to take them; still others were skeptical that something as unfamiliar as a global pandemic was really a threat to them and their family. We had to make clear to everyone what they needed to demand of their political leaders, and we had to address frontline health care workers about the challenges they were going to be facing.

One thing I felt sure of: people would be less likely to act unless they believed that other people would also act in a reasonably coordinated fashion. Getting that coordination would be hard for us to achieve from outside of government. As I wrote, the team began to work on the key elements of introducing the campaign to the country. I called my editor at *USA Today*, Jill Lawrence, and she agreed to publish the manifesto on March 16, 2020. *USA Today* is the most widely read publication in the country, with its articles syndicated to many local papers, reaching the broadest cross section of Americans: rich and poor, red and blue, rural and urban.

John and his colleague Alix Burns, an expert in messaging and communication, bought radio airtime in multiple languages in some of the hardest-hit areas of the country to get our key messages out to people who might not otherwise see them.

To reach younger people, John introduced me to the leaders of YouTube, who in turn introduced me to a number of YouTube creators with millions of younger subscribers. Reaching younger audiences was important because evidence was mounting that they were often among the first people in a community to get and spread the virus, but they were also less inclined to worry about getting sick from it.

At this time, influential people were already beginning to spread information to the public about flattening the curve, handwashing, social distancing, death tolls, and hospital workers. For the campaign to work best, I wanted to introduce a common language others could use. We created simple media talking points and a website where people could find resources and credible sources of information, and we made sure that we got them into the hands of the people who appeared most frequently as experts on cable TV.

Rob Bennett, a master of progressive online causes, lined up the forces of Twitter—celebrities, political activists, and other media influencers he knew.

Alix Burns developed a pitch for TV producers that she disseminated as soon as the story went up.

This would ultimately work only if we could spark citizen action and turn that into government action. Joanna Dornfeld, my colleague from United States of Care, took the manifesto and reworked it into a letter to send to all the governors and the mayors of the 50 largest cities in the nation. I prepared an email to send over to the White House when the time was right.

I invited a number of experts to review the draft, make comments, and sign on as supporters. Most of the voices on the topic—public health experts, Democrats and Republicans alike—thought we had it right. With their signatures, it became a show of force in public health. What we published was almost exactly what I wrote in my first draft. On March 15, it went up on the *USA Today* website:

The coronavirus pandemic seemed so far away just weeks ago.

No one likes to be isolated and sit at home and be bored.

You want to be near friends as you work from home.

The numbers you're hearing about the virus seem too big to believe.

You're worried about your neighbors and the impact on local businesses and workers.

You feel healthy, and how much worse can it be than the flu, after all?

COVID-19 is spreading, and you won't know you're infected until you've already infected others. Right now, you have no immunity to prevent you from getting the disease. It's especially lethal for older people or those with underlying conditions. This will come to communities in waves and will be a marathon, not a sprint, so pay attention to local events. And our hospitals won't have sufficient resources—people, beds, ventilators, or protective gear—if cases keep spreading as fast as they are in Italy.

But there's something important you can do: #StayHome.

STAY AT HOME as much as possible. It may be in your community now or it may be soon. Until you hear otherwise from health care officials, even if you have no symptoms. That means avoiding playdates, sleepovers, bars, restaurants, parties, and houses of worship. Avoid all crowds.

What can you do instead?

You can still take walks outside, shop for essentials, and enjoy your online community of friends.

Stay connected in other ways. Check in on your loved ones and friends frequently.

Keep informed about what is happening in your neighborhood.

Give to people in need in your community: supplies for food pantries, financial donations, personal hygiene items.

Buy online gift certificates to your favorite local stores and restaurants—and use them when this is over.

Be a neat freak. Keep everything as clean as possible.

Wash your hands. Early, often, thoroughly.

If you're going to spread anything, spread help, compassion, and humor.

Above all, do not panic. Remember: Like all outbreaks, this too will eventually end.

If you've been infected and recovered already, you are highly likely to be immune. If so, you can serve your community in public spaces where others can't.

To state and local leaders

Prioritize the most vulnerable in your community—the elderly, the sick, and those living in close quarters.

Temporarily close bars and restaurants when there is evidence of rising community transmission.

Work with Congress to provide continued economic support for your constituents most urgently affected by the pandemic's financial blow.

Consider temporary suspension of all commercial air and rail travel.

Ensure the safety and resources needed for your health care workforce. Health care and critical infrastructure workers should have the highest priority for personal protective equipment.

Make rapid expansion of COVID-19 testing a top priority. Open drive-through testing stations and offer at-home care.

Make prescription drug supply and other necessities in your community a priority.

Provide immediate training for all medical providers to join the effort wherever they can be most useful.

Honor cross-state medical licensing for all health care providers until the pandemic is over.

Prepare large spaces (stadiums, hotels) to become quarantine residences, as needed.

Coordinate with the National Guard to provide surge intensive-care-unit capacity for communities in need.

Create fever clinics for triage.

Reevaluate any regulations that impede the above (or below).

To health care workers

We know you are in uncharted waters and are standing on the front lines. All of us depend on your training, your compassion, your commitment, and your untapped capacity.

If you have not yet joined this fight, please reach out to your local hospital and find out how you can enlist.

Contact telemedicine platforms and offer your services.

Stop all elective surgical and medical procedures now.

Send people home if it's safest for them to be at home.

Reinforce the benefit of staying home and getting tested.

Help the people on the front lines do their jobs. Focused and united, we can avoid the worst possibilities. It's up to all of us. As a country, we can overcome this together.

#StayHome

www.stayhomesavelives.us

About two dozen well-recognized leaders put their name on the manifesto.[25]

Within the first week, 100 million people saw our #StayHome campaign. By the end of the year, it would reach nearly half a billion people. After we launched it, I made the rounds of cable TV to discuss it, and we got into deeper conversations with state and local officials. TV stations had gone from missing the story to nonstop coverage. They were beginning to discuss the possibility of taking unified action to control the virus's spread.

Not every point was heeded. Nursing homes, jails, public housing, and homeless shelters continued to have significant deaths; there was little evidence that they had become a priority for public officials. It wasn't until an early April story on Rachel Maddow's show on MSNBC that the public became fully aware of the terrible losses in nursing homes—but by then, tens of thousands had died.

Other recommendations were more successful. We started to see a larger swath of governors and mayors taking significant steps designed to save as many lives as possible, including temporarily shutting down places where the virus spread quickly. Hot spots like bars and restaurants—what New York City Council Speaker Corey Johnson had worried about earlier in March—would start to close quickly across the country. On March 19, 2020, California became the first state to issue a stay-at-home directive.[26] On March 21, Illinois and New Jersey followed. By March 23, nine states had. By March 26, 21 states had. And by March 30, a total of 30 states had issued some sort of stay-at-home order.[27]

The message to stay home, distance, and wear a mask—the most foreign of ideas—was becoming the norm in many places. At the same time, for some people, the manifesto and the state and local government stay-at-home orders that followed were overkill and an infringement on their liberty. While small initially, that group would grow larger and louder as time went on. And while similar concerns were relevant all over the world, the strength of that challenge was most striking in the United States.

To people like Bill Joy, on the other hand, the actions were helpful but insufficient. And he was right in this regard; the best time to take strong action was at the earliest point possible, before the public's patience wore thin.

There were some things to feel good about. Judging by Zach's math, the R0, or the virus's basic reproduction number, dropped rather quickly and seemingly miraculously from 2.3 to under 1.0 in most of the country in a manner of weeks.[28] The benefit was clear: more lives saved. According to a research study published in *Nature* in June, stay-at-home orders and social distancing that kept people from congregating prevented about 60 million novel coronavirus infections in the United States and tens of thousands of deaths.[29] Had we taken these steps weeks earlier, more lives would have been saved, but it wasn't possible to go back in time. *Save the next life*, I kept telling myself.

Saving lives from COVID-19 came with other costs. Mental

health issues and addiction, already at crisis levels before the pandemic, exploded. Family ties and friendships, which historically have gotten people through tough times, weren't as available or were cut off entirely. People living in nursing homes, assisted living, and our prison system faced unprecedented isolation from friends and family. The losses were many: the physical touch of a loved one, the stabilizing influence of schools, the disruptions to our favorite pastimes. Jobs were lost too, as large numbers of businesses found themselves without customers. These are huge costs, and they have caused the country to persistently ask: Is it worth it? It is important to keep these costs in mind as we continue to learn how to manage the threat from the virus.

But we didn't have to accept all these consequences as inevitable. A successful response was more of an orchestral performance than a solo act. Everyone would have to do their part to minimize the negative side effects of millions of people temporarily staying home. Congress had the ability to mitigate some of these issues with financial support and messages of assurance to the public. In Germany, the government provided financial support to the bars and restaurants that closed to keep the public safe. There was no reason we couldn't do that here—and increase public support and trust in the government at the same time. Public support led to much better compliance. Encouraging the federal government to step up to address these side effects became a big part of the work we had to do, but as I will cover in Chapter 4, support from Republicans waned as it became clearer that the duration of the pandemic would be longer than they had hoped.

The economic consequences of agreeing to temporarily freeze elements of the economy were an important issue. Many assert without good evidence that the stay-at-home orders were the cause of financial hardship. Evidence suggests that it's the virus, not the shutdown, that is the real culprit in economic downturns. During the 1918 flu pandemic, those cities with swifter, more robust responses to the pandemic had the most rapidly improving economies.[30] The same appears to be true with COVID-19. Actions taken to save lives didn't cause the economic crisis, as some have tried to portray.[31] Quite the opposite, in fact. Those countries with strong responses—Vietnam, Hong Kong, South Korea, and New Zealand—were able to contain the virus faster and put in place policies to ensure safe openings. These countries' economies have thus far fared the best.[32]

But economic analyses like this oversimplify the reality. Yes, many of the big things that drive the economy—large consumer purchases such as cars and vacations; business spending on machinery, new leases, and hiring; and foreign trade—would be unlikely to recover with the pandemic raging. But if you ask a bar owner to temporarily close for 60 days and the owner only has 30 days of cash in the bank, analyses from 1918 don't much matter. Our national conscience needed to extend to all kinds of pain.

Getting the President's Attention

My family and I were going through the same process of figuring out how to alter our habits and routines as everybody else. On March 11, we'd canceled long-standing plans to celebrate Lana's birthday at a local Minneapolis restaurant. As everyone else stayed home, rumors of shortages turned into real shortages of things like flour, sugar, soap, and toilet paper. We made sure we were stocked up, but not with more than our share. It was strange to see shelves start to empty. Soon Lana was sewing masks and sending them, along with hand sanitizer and other needed items, to friends and family who were having difficulty finding what they needed. Someone on Twitter offered to drive a roll of toilet paper to my house if I ever needed it; fortunately, I never faced that kind of jam.

I asked myself, for the first time, whether I was worried for us. Lana is a breast cancer survivor and has some immune system issues. Our older son, Caleb, had childhood asthma. Our younger son, Zach, experiences a bout with pneumonia almost every winter. I was in reasonably good health but was 53. I also have epilepsy, which was a risk factor if I got COVID-19, but I was more concerned about running out of the medication I take to manage it. All things considered, I felt like we were damned lucky compared to many people.

On March 17, as I relaxed in front of the television, I heard the news anchor announce that the United States had hit 100 deaths from COVID-19. With Zach's math in mind, I typed out a tweet: "100 death mark today, we will cross the mark where hundreds, then thousands will join this list. Keep the people you love at home. Please."[33]

So much depended on whether President Trump decided to join the fight. Procuring testing, getting equipment to hospitals, supporting displaced businesses, building out the surge capacity of hospitals—all relied on the full weight of the federal government and the military. None of that could happen without the president. How could we get through to him?

In New York City, Anthony Scaramucci was wondering the same thing. Scaramucci, famous for his 11-day stint as White House communications director in the summer of 2017, has a reputation for being brash, self-promoting, and outspoken, and he is all of that. But a less well-known side of him is that he is extremely well-read, is an avid student of history, and has deep insight into the mindset of one Donald J. Trump.

He described to me what he thought was causing Trump not to act in the face of an obvious crisis and what eventually might convince him to change his mind. To understand Trump, he told me, you need to understand that he will always do what he believes is best for himself. "Where we are is, he did not want to close that economy, because when you're thinking about T-R-U-M-P closing the economy, you're gonna have growth slippage, you're going to have higher unemployment. His whole narrative is, and he says this at his rallies, 'You may hate me, but you like your 401(k) and you like the economy and you like where the stock market is. And so you're gonna vote for me anyway.' That's his narrative.

"So when someone comes in and says, 'Hey, the South Koreans are shutting down their economy, they have experience with MERS and SARS and we're gonna go into a 21- or 28-day lockdown and that's actually going to save the economy,' he's like . . . 'I'm not going to go in that direction, okay?'

"And now he's getting pounded," Scaramucci continued. "Then he does a lot of press conferences. And what President Trump tries to do is he tries to curve reality towards his version of reality. And [historically] he's been very successful in doing that.

"But not this time. Throughout his career, Trump's best tools were controlling the narrative, presenting an image of himself as in control, bullying and provoking, going against the grain to get attention, blaming others, and if all else fails, declaring bankruptcy and leaving someone else holding the bag. But those tools, which had won him tens of millions of supporters in his run for the presidency, and which he used to fend off Democrats and the establishment, didn't work against . . . immutable forces like a virus."[34]

They didn't work with Wall Street traders either. On Thursday, March 12, the Dow dropped 2,352 points, a 10 percent plunge—the worst day since Black Monday in 1987. The following Monday, the day our manifesto was published, it dropped another 12 percent, the third-worst drop in market history. For Trump, this was now a real crisis.

Scaramucci told me that on the weekend following the March 12 sell-off, "a couple of very senior guys from Wall Street met with him" and told him if he didn't act on the virus, "you're going to have hundreds of thousands of people die. And you're going to have a nightmare in the economy."

On the night of March 16, after I finished a TV interview about the #StayHome campaign and sat down with Lana for a cocktail, my phone rang. It was two staffers from the White House.

"Finally," I mouthed to Lana, who looked at me quizzically.

They were putting together a set of social distancing guidelines for the president to introduce, and sent over a draft for me to look at. They pulled up a copy of the *USA Today* manifesto, and the three of us walked through how to work it into guidelines the president could release.

When I got off the call, I sank down in my chair and let my shoulders relax for the first time in quite a while. I sent John, Alix, and the rest of the team a note of thanks and took a few long, deep breaths.

On the morning of Tuesday, March 17, the president announced at a press briefing that for the next 15 days, "we're asking everyone to work at home, if possible, postpone unnecessary travel, and limit social gatherings to no more than 10 people. By making shared sacrifices and temporary changes, we can protect the health of our people and we can protect our economy, because I think our economy will come back very rapidly."[35] Of course, 15 days wouldn't be nearly enough. But #StayHome had penetrated the walls of the White House.

CHAPTER 4

THE VIRUS AND THE WHITE HOUSE, PART I

SCENE: THE HALLS OF POWER, WASHINGTON, D.C.

> If you need to be right before you move, you will never win. Perfection is the enemy of the good when it comes to emergency management. Speed trumps perfection. And the problem with society that we have at the moment is that everyone is afraid of making a mistake. . . . But the gravest error is not to move. The gravest error is to be paralyzed by the fear of failure. And I think that's the single biggest lesson I've learned in Ebola responses in the past.
>
> —Dr. Michael Ryan, executive director of the WHO Health Emergencies Programme, March 13, 2020[1]

The stock market plunge was not the only worry at the White House. The man leading the pandemic task force, Alex Azar, the secretary of Health and Human Services and a former executive with the pharmaceutical company Eli Lilly, oversaw a series of unforced errors. For Trump, tired of all the negative press, HHS's mistakes added to an already strained relationship with Azar.

From the start, embarrassing failures plagued HHS. Most notably, the CDC made a series of costly stumbles. The most important thing they needed to do was to create enough diagnostic tests to locate and contain outbreaks and quarantine anyone infected. The CDC decided to use its own test, rather than one developed by the WHO. It wasn't an unusual decision, but it added to the time the virus could circulate before anyone infected could be identified and asked to isolate. But they made a less publicized yet more detrimental decision. With the coronavirus knocking at our door, the major commercial and academic laboratories had begun working almost immediately on their own diagnostic tests, gearing up to blanket the country with them. Labs approached the CDC in early February and offered to develop a test that could be rolled out quickly. But on February 20, HHS sent out an email blast saying that the CDC's test would be the only one authorized by the FDA, and only a hand-picked set of labs with limited capacity would be allowed to use it. The FDA, like the CDC, is part of HHS. Both report to Azar.

Lab directors were incredulous. Diagnostic testing was the only way to detect an invisible virus. In contrast, South Korea, which had its first reported case on January 19, the same day as the United States, harnessed the power of its clinical laboratories and manufacturers and in less than three weeks its version of the CDC and FDA had certified tests from 46 different nongovernment laboratories.[2] As physician and author Atul Gawande noted, South Korea also implemented a uniform price and a uniform text-based scheduling system, putting access to a test and rapid results within reach of everyone.[3] Our failure in getting enough tests manufactured early in the pandemic cost us our single opportunity to get on South Korea's curve and keep the virus contained.

But at least we had the test the CDC developed, right? Except soon after its launch, reports started coming in that part of the CDC test was contaminated. I began receiving calls from state health officials, including from North Carolina, telling me that the test the CDC developed didn't work.[4] Meanwhile, Vice President Mike

Pence was on TV crowing about the "tens of thousands" of tests available even after it was well known to labs and hospitals across the country that the tests were useless.[5]

The CDC's testing failure was huge. But, sadly, it was a small part of a bigger problem. There was no unified crisis strategy being followed throughout HHS, and the lack of trust and coordination between Secretary Azar and some of the people who ran the agencies within HHS was part of the problem. Azar had decided not to include anyone from the FDA or CMS in the ad hoc task force he created on January 11, 2020. This was despite the critical roles these agencies needed to play in the pandemic response: the FDA to approve tests, therapies, and vaccines and CMS to agree to pay for whatever the FDA approved and to protect seniors in nursing homes.

Out of the daily loop of the task force, the FDA was working at its normal, careful pace. It is designed to be a deliberative and measured body and to protect the public from poor quality, not to respond quickly to an exponentially spreading pathogen. That approach fit right in with the administration's tone of not sounding the alarm too loudly.

My experience in large-scale national crises has taught me to never put all your eggs in one basket, but to create several different paths to success. That way, if you make mistakes—and you are bound to make them—no single mistake is catastrophic. Prohibiting the nation's laboratories from rolling out their own tests violated every strategic rule for crisis management. This is precisely the kind of error that could have been avoided if the playbook created by Ebola Task Force head Ron Klain during the Obama administration had been followed.

Azar, who has described himself as one of the country's leading experts on pandemic preparedness, faulted the FDA and said he never knew about their decision not to allow outside labs to create their own tests; the people at the FDA blamed Azar and said they sought permission to work with external labs but were turned down, in order to stay consistent with the White House's efforts to play down the virus. Even if Azar had been surprised, he did not correct the decision for a long time. Azar knew that visibility into where and how fast the virus was moving was his number one priority, and he didn't have any visibility. And he did not warn the public.

The King's Yes-Men

These failures marked the collapse of the country's first line of defense. The missed opportunity to contain the virus early had lasting consequences. In many respects, the course of the virus and its impact on Americans were determined at the moment diagnostic tests could not be manufactured while the number of infected people was still low. The implications were profound. Soon thousands of tests would not suffice; we would need tens of millions. Now, with no way to detect the virus, the public would have to assume everyone they came into contact with was potentially infectious. All the burden of preventing its spread would need to be shifted from the scientists to the public in the form of mask wearing, remaining physically distant, and staying home. This single failure ultimately led to closing schools, restaurants, gyms, barbershops, sports arenas, and on and on. Most disturbingly, Trump, Pence, and Azar never warned the public of this reality, stripping Americans of the ability to mount a second line of defense.

The lack of a coherent testing strategy cannot be pinned solely on Azar. With the president of the United States on TV saying the virus was a hoax and the White House communications team breathing down Azar's neck, how could the HHS secretary tell every lab in the country to respond at crisis levels?

Trump had appointed Azar in 2017 at Mike Pence's recommendation. Azar replaced Tom Price, who had resigned under pressure after allegations of corruption and who had been disliked by just about everybody. Azar had formerly served at HHS as general counsel and as deputy secretary and had clerked for Supreme Court justice Antonin Scalia before becoming an executive at Eli Lilly. While

at HHS, Azar had been deeply involved in pandemic preparation under George W. Bush and HHS secretary Mike Leavitt. In late 2017,
after Trump nominated him, Azar asked my advice on his Senate
confirmation hearing. He was anxious not to join education secretary Betsy DeVos as the only cabinet member who had not received
a single confirmation vote from the opposition party.

"Alex, as far as Democrats are concerned, you're definitely not
the worst possible choice," I told him at the time. "Personally, I like
the fact that you have respect for the career staff and don't buy
into that deep-state garbage."

I knew Alex and I weren't going to see eye to eye on most policy
issues, as would be the case with any Trump appointee. Before I spoke
about him to the Democratic senators, though, I had one question:
"What happens when you're in the room with Trump and he says
something dumb or irresponsible? Will you have the political capital to protect your equities? Democrats need to be convinced you
are willing to get into the argument and have the capital to win
with Trump."

He tried to assuage my concerns. "The president and I talked
about this. And he knows I'm of strong will."

Azar won confirmation with yea votes from five Democratic
senators.

Despite having a deep conceptual understanding of how to respond to a pandemic, when COVID-19 hit, Azar had only a tenu-
ous grip on the department, and his credibility in the White House
had been damaged both by the CDC's test manufacturing debacle
and by Trump's anger at the bad press he continually received on
health care.

Unlike most other cabinet departments, HHS is structured with
a number of strong, highly independent agencies underneath it.
The four biggest are the Centers for Medicare and Medicaid Services, the Food and Drug Administration, the National Institutes
of Health, and the Centers for Disease Control and Prevention. In
fairness to Azar, the heads of these agencies historically run them
autonomously and have fairly independent public profiles. It was

practically a rule that the four agencies rarely communicated, as they were located in different parts of the country and had very different missions and cultures. HHS has had some great leaders, including my old boss Sylvia Burwell, but unlike the roles of secretaries in other cabinet departments who directly oversaw day-to-day poli-cymaking and operations, the HHS secretary's role often amounted to oversight of the agencies and being something of a speechmaker and a go-between with the White House or Congress.

Azar had difficult working relationships with many of the de-partment's most important leaders and principal White House staff. For most of 2019, he fought a very public battle with Seema Verma, who succeeded me at CMS.[6] Though it's not clear how the feud started, before long Azar or his surrogates were leaking in-formation about Verma, and Verma about Azar. It seemed to close observers that one of them would have to go. Since they were both from Indiana, the vice president brought them together for a sit-down in the White House on the afternoon of December 11, 2019. At that meeting, Verma told Pence she would stay only if she wouldn't be required to work with Azar any longer (normally the secretary was required to sign off on the CMS administra-tor's decisions). In an embarrassment to Azar, Pence agreed.[7] With Azar's standing already low, after the mishaps with the pandemic the White House staff met to consider replacing him as HHS secre-tary. Trump had given a directive that no one would be fired from the health team during the pandemic. Even still, a senior White House official told me it was a close decision not to fire Azar and replace him with Verma.

Left to his own, Azar understood much of what was needed to respond to the pandemic. But his boss did not. Cabinet secretar-ies aren't supposed to just go along with the president when they disagree. The HHS secretary is supposed to make sure health care is delivered to more than 100 million people, federal investments are made in medical research, the nation has a safe and adequate drug supply, public health is protected, and we are prepared for disasters. But Azar needed to please a man who had little interest in those goals and little more than disdain for the tens of thousands of men and women working to achieve them.

On January 3, Azar received an email from CDC director Redfield about a flu-like illness in Wuhan that they had become aware of on New Year's Eve. The first report was of 25 patients. As Azar learned more, he notified then–chief of staff Mick Mulvaney and Bob O'Brien, the national security advisor. Trump was apparently notified in his next Presidential Daily Briefing. But two and a half months would pass before the White House finally mounted a response. On January 11, Azar convened a task force, which included Anthony Fauci from the NIH; Robert Redfield; and Robert Kadlec, the HHS assistant secretary in charge of emergency response. But in an unusual and costly decision, he did not include FDA commissioner Stephen Hahn or CMS administrator Seema Verma.

Azar briefed Trump by phone for the first time on January 18, 2020, while Trump was at Mar-a-Lago. Azar wasn't aiming to alarm the president; in fact, his primary goal was to make sure the president was prepared in case he received questions from reporters on his trip to the World Economic Forum in Davos, Switzerland. Azar conveyed to the president that HHS currently had things under control. Was it a standard reassurance? Was it an expression of overconfidence? Either way, the president's reaction was matter-of-fact and, even though Azar underplayed the new disease's potential to cause problems in the United States, Trump still thought he was being alarmist.[8]

A president who was uninterested in details and wanted to minimize bad news was a bad match for a secretary he didn't trust and who was trying to improve his standing with his boss. If anyone could have seen the potential death toll, it was Azar. What he should have done that first day in January was what Nancy Messonnier did a month later—tell the public to prepare for the coming crisis.

Azar was part of an administration whose culture rewarded yesmen and publicly humiliated anyone brave enough to acknowledge difficult truths. Nobody wanted to experience what Messonnier had. And Azar even participated in harshly criticizing her for stepping out of line.[9] It would have required significant personal courage for Azar to speak out. Instead he clung to his job.

Azar was formally the chair of the pandemic task force, which had a total of 12 members. But Azar wasn't in control; instead, O'Brien's deputy national security advisor, Matthew Pottinger, or White House chief of staff Mick Mulvaney ran the meetings in the White House Situation Room. But the focus of the meetings was not on core elements of pandemic response—creating new testing, replenishing the depleted supply of PPE and other supplies, preparing the health care system or the public—but instead on figuring out how to extract American citizens from China and on ineffective efforts at border control. There was no preparation for what would happen if the borders were breached. And even the measures they did take were bound to be ineffective. By the time Trump acted to restrict travel, 300,000 people had traveled to the United States from China during January alone.[10] Efforts to close down travel from Europe were reportedly blocked by treasury secretary Steve Mnuchin. Azar's request for funds to buy more PPE was opposed by Joe Grogan, a principal aide to Mulvaney who had frequently clashed with Azar, and budget officials; they cut it by 40 percent. All the while, the global supply chain for those items shrank.

Azar was removed as head of the Coronavirus Task Force on February 26 and replaced with Mike Pence. The White House Task Force meetings continued in the Situation Room, located on the lower level of the West Wing. But there was something noticeably odd about them. They were, in effect, senior HHS department meetings—only chaired by Pence and without the department head himself. Instead, Hahn and Verma were now invited. Inviting agency heads into the Situation Room with the vice president and without their boss certainly sent a clear message to Azar. But it was also a bad dynamic. People such as Hahn, who had been in government only a short time, were described as "starry-eyed" and eager to oblige requests from the VP. Not only was the pandemic out of Azar's hands; so was the department. And he was prohibited from speaking to the press. (And you think your office is dysfunctional.)

In Barack Obama's White House, false confidence did not go over well. Telling the president you had things under control if you didn't was taboo. And while you always wanted to deliver the goods for the president, overpromising was a bad idea. The president and his team, led by chief of staff Denis McDonough, expected an honest conversation about risks. Entering the second year of Obamacare, after that first traumatic year, I was tasked by Secretary Burwell with briefing Obama on whether the second year would be better than the first. In our first briefing on the topic, the president asked me if the health insurance exchanges would launch successfully and on time. Rather than say yes, I provided a brief rundown of what we were doing to make it happen, and my confidence level on a scale of 1 to 100. Each time I updated him, I would update that assessment. The second year went off virtually without a hitch; even still, whenever there was any issue—even if the website was down for just five minutes—we informed the White House.

Obama, furthermore, wanted the recommendations we gave him separated from the politics. I mentioned to him once that a recommendation I made likely wouldn't go over well politically, even with his supporters.

"The politics are my job. Just tell me what you think the right thing to do is," he said. "And then do it. I will deal with the politics."

Trump, on the other hand, loved yes-men, and he got them. When he pushed the FDA to approve the drug hydroxychloroquine as a COVID-19 treatment despite a lack of scientific evidence, the agency obliged. When Trump wanted to announce a 100-year-old therapy called convalescent plasma as if it were a "scientific breakthrough," Azar and his team did not stand in the way; not only that, they appeared on billboards promoting it. In the fall, Azar went so far as to revoke the requirement that the FDA review tests developed in independent labs, thus removing a crucial safeguard; it was exactly what he should have done in January, but not in October.[11] In a bid to show loyalty to a president who wanted to wield control over the FDA, he took the even more unusual step of not allowing the FDA to issue regulations any longer, taking that authority for himself. None of those moves had any precedent in anyone's memory.

Academy Award–winning director Alex Gibney, who interviewed many of the people in HHS for a documentary he was filming called *Totally Under Control*, told me that after all the threatening and firing and ostracizing, Trump now had a set of people who told him "only what he wanted to hear, not what he needed to hear."

Trump Spins the Virus Response

One political appointee from the Obama administration stayed on under Trump—my friend David Shulkin, who became secretary of veterans affairs. Shulkin, a doctor from New Jersey, had been undersecretary of the Department of Veterans Affairs (VA) for Obama. When I first met him in 2010, he was the CEO of a nonprofit hospital in New Jersey, and he was eminently qualified for the real work needed to make care better in the VA, even if he wasn't as expert at navigating the politics of the Trump administration. Like Jim Mattis, the secretary of defense, Shulkin viewed Trump with a wary eye, but he thought he could provide service in this extraordinary moment and act to protect the VA against some of Trump's worst instincts. Within months, though, Trump had placed a number of his friends and campaign donors around Shulkin to watch him and vet every decision, just as he'd done with Redfield at the CDC. Shulkin didn't last long in the Trump administration (nor did Mattis).

One evening early in his tenure as secretary, I was in D.C. and Shulkin invited me over to his apartment to talk about a presentation he was going to make to Trump.

"You wouldn't believe this guy," Shulkin said. "He promises the world and there's no possible way to deliver it."

Trump had pledged during his campaign to dismantle the VA and allow veterans to get care from anywhere they wanted. But there were too many veterans with too many needs for that to be possible, nor would Congress allow it. Shulkin also understood there were a host of areas in which the VA has unique expertise, from post-traumatic stress to limb prosthetics. Besides, veterans and veterans' groups loved the VA; they just wanted to see it improved. So Trump's proposals, while ideologically appealing to his donors, were impractical. A law passed during the Obama administration (for which Trump took credit) did give veterans the choice to get care outside the VA. But Trump wanted Shulkin to deliver something close to full privatization.

Shulkin said, "When I tell him we can't deliver, I think he's going to go ballistic."

"I have a feeling this is nothing like briefing Obama," I replied.

"I expect you're right."

I knew other people who had presented to Trump. Zeke Emanuel, an oncologist and bioethicist who had worked at the National Institutes of Health since 1997 and in the first two years of the Obama administration, had repeatedly pleaded the case to Trump not to repeal the ACA just after the election and in the first few months of 2017. Emanuel had told me the formula for a successful presentation.

"Begin the meeting with two compliments," he'd said. "If you do that, it's going to go well. My problem is I only have two 'compliments' for Trump, so I've had to use them three times. 'Mr. President, you have such excellent kids. It is clear you are a great father.' 'Mr. President, you have done an amazing job restoring the Trump Hotel from the Old Post Office in D.C.'" After the two compliments, Trump always responded with how smart the complimenter was.

Shulkin and I discussed his plans to increase choice for veterans and to create more pressure for the VA hospitals to improve their performance. Both ideas were quite reasonable and had the support of Congress and the major veterans' groups.

"Why don't you say this: 'Mr. President, you've promised a 10. I can deliver a 4 that we can dress up as a 6,'" I suggested.

Shulkin smiled. He liked it and decided to use it. After the briefing, he told me it had worked.

"What did he say?"

"He thought for a moment and said, 'That would take a heck of a marketing job.'"

"And you said?"

"'Mr. President, I think you can do it.' And he thought for a minute and I wasn't sure where he was going. Finally he says, 'Can you make it a 7?' And I realized he thought we were having a negotiation. So I pretended to think about it for a minute and said, 'Yes, we can do that,' as if I had actually changed anything in substance."

Trump was all about the presentation. For him, perception was reality. After a series of ups and downs in his business career, Trump wasn't so much in real estate any longer as he was increasingly franchising his name to partners who did the real work. He realized that for a fee and less risk, he could put his name on a building, a necktie, some steaks, or a university. His job was to keep the value of the brand up and let the money flow in. Trump's businesses were mostly about publicity, cash, and royalties. R&D, strategic planning, and the many other functions in business besides marketing and the dark arts of leverage were completely foreign to Trump.

With its hand forced by the stock market's declines, the White House began taking action. On March 12, Jared Kushner enlisted Adam Boehler to lead a team to finally address what the task force had ignored—locating ventilators, buying PPE, and other logistical matters. Boehler, who at the time was overseeing the U.S. International Development Finance Corporation, was a friend of mine, a successful entrepreneur, apolitical, and the kind of person you want on your team during a crisis. The team Kushner and Boehler built consisted largely of New York investment bankers, consultants, and people who worked in private equity firms. Forty was considered old for this group; most were in their thirties, had never been in government, and had never run anything big. That made them a target of media scoffing, but the people they recruited were smart, capable volunteers entirely willing to put their lives on hold and work 100-hour weeks under less-than-ideal circumstances. I was glad they were there, and I sent a few additional talented people their way.

With the stock market still dropping, Trump arranged a big press conference where Kushner, Boehler, and Nat Turner, also a friend of mine and a successful health care entrepreneur, could help him put on a show of force.

On March 13, the CEOs of Walgreens, Walmart, Roche, Abbott, and Target stood behind Trump as he announced grand plans, including hundreds of drive-through testing sites at pharmacies and retailers as well as a website to be produced by Google, where people could go to check symptoms and find a testing site if warranted. "Stores in virtually every location. Google has 1,700 engineers working on this right now," he said.[12]

It all sounded good. But it wasn't true.

The new White House team had only just started to work. They'd had a preliminary call with a senior executive in one of Google Alphabet's divisions, in which they'd requested help building a website, but they had been short on specifics. In an emergency, good people are inclined to say yes first and ask questions later. So this executive agreed and handed the assignment off to a small team, but the White House hadn't even figured out what they needed. The Google team called me the next weekend to ask for my ideas on what to build. I did not envy them.

In the end, the White House team decided that the national drive-through testing program and tracking website weren't great ideas after a three-hour line at a state-run drive-through testing site in Denver generated bad publicity.[13]

The White House team wasn't entirely to blame here. They made one mistake however: they told the president what they were working on before they had figured out how to do it. With more time, these details might have been worked out, or the initial ideas scrapped for a better plan. But with the stock market tanking, Trump the showman needed something for his show. Part of a staff member's job, though, is to protect a president against his worst instincts, not feed them, as happened here.

In this case, Trump got what he wanted out of his press conference, even if the American public didn't. That day saw the single biggest rise in the stock market's history, making up a portion of the ground that had been lost. Trump celebrated this win with the team, although it had the unfortunate effect of removing the pressure on him to actually do something real to combat the virus. The stock market, not the death toll, was his measure of success. Trump was so pleased he had reprints made of the newspaper headline showing the stock market's record rise, signed them, framed them, and gave them as gifts to the team that brought the press conference together. With the stock market now rising, for him the crisis was effectively over.

The Easter Sunday Massacre

Trump did not like what "the doctors" (as the White House economic staff derisively called Anthony Fauci and Deborah Birx) were telling him about how bad the virus was and the need for strict, sustained action. Richard Epstein was not a doctor. Nor was he an epidemiologist, virologist, statistician, or data scientist. He was a law professor who authored papers on topics like why it's okay to deny care to poor people and why poor people should be permitted to sell their organs to the highest bidder.[14] He was a libertarian. When COVID-19 began, Epstein was pretty sure he could predict what would happen when the pandemic came to the United States.[15] On March 16, 2020, he published a paper in which he decried use of the label "pandemic," suggesting the virus was no worse than the flu and estimated that America's death toll would be no greater than 500 people. He called higher estimates "hysterical and sloppy," and claimed stay-at-home measures "have wrecked both the economy and upended the lives of millions of people." A week later, as the death toll rose, he surreptitiously edited the paper to increase the estimate of deaths to 5,000 and claimed the previous number had been an error.[16] After hearing about Epstein's predictions, Donald Trump had found what he needed—one "expert" whose opinions he could use to justify his actions. On March 22, Trump tweeted, in his signature all-caps style, "WE CANNOT LET THE CURE BE WORSE THAN THE PROBLEM ITSELF."[17]

(I debated Epstein a few months later and found him to be both disconnected from reality and remarkably self-assured. He was supposed to be defending President Trump in the debate, but instead he spent much of his time attacking critics of hydroxychloroquine, speculating on new theories of why the death toll couldn't possibly be real, and suggesting that the virus would only last two months if we just let people get sick. All of those, incidentally, were things we heard from Trump's lips at some point.[18])

By March 23, stay-at-home orders had been implemented in nine states.[19] #StayHome was everywhere—it was taking root on lawn signs and in common vernacular—but we knew it would be two to three weeks before we'd see the results of our actions, as the presymptomatic period and test result lags meant there was no instant gratification. The hard part of this pandemic was to stay confident that you were on the right course in the absence of immediate data.

On March 24, in an interview on Fox News a week after Epstein's paper was published, Trump made a statement that threatened to derail everything we had begun. "Easter's a very special day for me," he said. "And I say, wouldn't it be great to have all of the churches full? I think Easter Sunday, you'll have packed churches all around the country."[20]

By my estimation, on Easter, the country would be beginning to reduce the rate of daily infections. But Trump wanted people around the country—including older, higher-risk churchgoers—to come together to pack the pews elbow to elbow and sing. By the end of April, our crisis would multiply.

Easter was in 18 days. Trump's comments sent the message to the country that we were almost done, when in fact we were only just starting. Much of the world was either on lockdown or playing it very safe. Countries with far fewer cases hadn't opened up yet. On March 18, German chancellor Angela Merkel said, "*Es ist ernst*"—the situation is serious, take it seriously. She went on to say that "since German unification—no, since the Second World War—no challenge to our nation has ever demanded such a degree of common and united action."[21] That same day, Donald Trump referred to himself as a "wartime president."[22]

At the time, only Trump's inner circle and the journalist Bob Woodward, who had been conducting on-the-record interviews with the president in preparation for a book, knew that Trump was aware of the massive tragedy about to befall the country. Unlike most people who comment on Trump, I wasn't consumed with the need to understand his motives. Most things about the president weren't going to change: the disorganization, the distrust of expertise, the overreliance on instinct, the avoidance of bad news, and, of course, the lying. But we had to get him to give up on an Easter opening. It would save tens of thousands of lives.

I needed to find someone to talk to. The answer to almost every question as to who was in charge at the White House, to one degree or another, was Jared Kushner. He was the one consistent influence on the president. People who wanted to make inroads in the White House went through Kushner.

I called someone outside the White House who I knew spoke with Kushner regularly and asked them to convey a simple message: "I know how hard this is from the inside and I'm happy to help." I was telling the truth. I had experienced crises during my time in government. The media follows your every move. You don't have time to think. You have limited staff. You don't get any breaks, and the bad news keeps coming. And that's if you're doing it well.

In a real crisis, there's no version of "I can deliver a 4 you can dress up like a 6." The 4 looks like a 4 very quickly. And with Trump there was no intellectual debate or discussion of the impact of his policies on real people. There was only the question of whether he was personally impacted.

The next day, I was sitting in the kitchen talking to Lana when Kushner's name came across my iPhone screen. He was courteous and friendly, soft-spoken, and gracious. He thanked me for some of the help I was providing. In turn, I offered to help further.

"We should all be putting politics aside. As long as we have lives to save, you should have the support of everybody in the country," I told him.

"I agree, thank you. And I'm a Democrat in a sea of Republicans," he said. I didn't know if this described his general reality or whether he was just trying to show me that we could be on the same side of things.

He told me how he thought about the pandemic: "There are three phases. There's the panic phase, the pain phase, and then the comeback phase. We are past the panic and about to move past the pain. It won't be entirely gone, but we now have to lead the comeback phase." The next month he shared a similar perspective in an interview with Bob Woodward.[23]

These phases—panic, pain, comeback—were a little too neat. More important, they were just a political construct, not something a virus would pay attention to. Still, I echoed his language and suggested that while we had an opportunity to reduce the pain phase, we couldn't accomplish that if we tried to get past it too hastily.

We moved on to cover other topics, and he told me about their progress in finding PPE and ventilators. I was glad for any positive news, late or not. But it was hard for me to fully calibrate how much progress was being made from an administration that only reported positive news and no benchmarks. The administration was largely successful in locating ventilators. (After Adam Boehler created a system to deliver ventilators as they were needed, I did agree later to tweet the availability of the program. The unusual part of the request is that after I tweeted about it, Ivanka Trump retweeted me.)

I got to the point of the call. "I think we need to change direction on Easter. It would be a big mistake." I went on to explain my reasoning: "Look, I think our metrics for opening up should be milestone-based, not time-based. Just like the president wouldn't position the exit from Afghanistan only on the basis of a date, he should also make this withdrawal one that is conditions-based. Challenge the country to deliver specific results so we can get back our lives. Be hopeful, but ask for sacrifice."

Kushner was listening and didn't seem to object. I offered another, more political thought: "The other benefit to him is he can point to the governors and the states and push them to reach those metrics. If he opens on a specific day like Easter, I think he gets all the blame when things go badly."

"Makes sense. Can you send me a paper that outlines how this would work?"

"Yes, I can get you something. But I suggest you get some from others so you can find a consensus," I said. I was confident that any public health professional would tell him the same thing. I suggested Scott Gottlieb, the former FDA commissioner, who I knew was putting together a paper on this topic as well.

"I'm talking to Scott later in the week."

"Great."

The Brain Trust

When I got off the phone with Kushner, I called John Doerr. He was deeply worried about the Easter Sunday announcement. We agreed it was a lot of additional deaths just to have a sound bite.

"Can we put a public paper together describing why opening on Easter Sunday would be bad?" John asked.

"I think we can do better." I relayed my conversation with Kushner and told John, "I need some help."

"We can collect the best scientific minds to come up with a plan. Do you want to call Bill Joy?"

I hesitated for a second. Bill would want to emulate the hard lockdown of Wuhan in our pandemic response. Drastic solutions would not convince the president to budge from his position. Still, I agreed we should include him.

"We at least need to get the president to delay," I said. I was standing and pacing, staring at my slippers, not even able to fully register the absurdity of Trump opening churches on Easter Sunday.

"And what about Larry Brilliant? He's the scientist who helped eradicate smallpox, and he was the pandemic advisor on the movie *Contagion*," John suggested. I agreed, and John set up a call with the four of us in an hour.

Some days, since the pandemic began, I would be eating like a 14-year-old boy and drinking like a 70-year-old man: ham and cheese quesadillas and smoothies during the day and a glass of wine or a cocktail at night, though rarely more than one. *Maybe I could learn some bartending skills*, I thought idly. I was better at imagining self-improvement projects than actually doing them, but now wasn't quite the right time to start: every day was a torrent of new activity. I wasn't feeling stress, just adrenaline at all there was to do.

When it came time for the call with John, Bill, and Larry, it was evening and I was in the front yard with our puppy, Brodie, trying to keep him from digging holes and eating mulch.

"I think the right plan is to buy time," I explained to Larry and Bill while Brodie hunted for spots that met his standards for relieving himself. "Give Trump a political out. Devise a system for reopening that is conditions-based, not time-based."

"Killing fewer people is still killing people," Bill said. He sounded crankier than ever about my half-measures. As I had expected, he still believed that only a Wuhan-style lockdown would suffice.

"We're not choosing between doing the right thing and doing the wrong thing," I said. "We are undoubtedly choosing between two wrong things—one better, one worse." The whole pandemic was mostly a series of not-so-good choices.

John, who had assumed the role of facilitator on this call, asked

Larry, "What do you think?" John did not like to overstep his expertise. He had achieved what he had not by believing he was the smartest person in the room but by finding the smartest people for the room.

If Bill was unbending, Larry had the presence of a sage or mystic. "What Andy said makes sense. We will need to convene the right experts to figure out the milestones." He knew who needed to be involved, and he kindly offered to help.

Addressing Bill specifically, Larry added, "We need national security thinking. Relative risks, not all-or-nothing measures." He had a way of saying things that made them profound yet obvious— like Yoda. ("No perfect pandemic response will there be, Andy.")

Bill sighed. He sounded angry. He didn't like this. Fifteen years of predicting doom only to finally be facing it but not being listened to—it was getting to him. Larry matched Bill's frustration with equal measures of calm and assurances that he understood. But Bill was always going to be the birdie on my shoulder—I would hear him everywhere I went, urging me to push for the strongest actions possible.

"Tell me again why we should do anything to support Trump," Bill said. A fair point.

"This isn't to help Trump. It's to help the people who don't have to die," I answered. "That's all we can do."

He got it. He didn't like it, but he got it.

"If Andy can get this to the president or Jared, let's put this together," John said, and began writing down the names of experts who Larry believed could give us useful input.

Larry sent an email introduction to several people in which he invited them to participate in a call and told them we were "looking for three or four punchy Trumpian bullet points to be walked into, talked into, President Trump to avert an Easter Sunday massacre if he actually would tell the entire country to stop social distancing and 'get back to work.'" From then on, we only referred to this event as the Easter Sunday Massacre.

One of the recipients of Larry's email was Baruch Fischhoff, a distinguished professor at Carnegie Mellon. Fischhoff is an expert on decision-making under risk, and he helped me understand what we were up against. In his view, the core issues we needed to address were at least as much psychological and behavioral as scientific. Fischhoff's view is that people care much more about their own lives than about statistics on infections and deaths. If people aren't feeling safe, that supersedes anything else. He was foreshadowing a problem that would emerge in the coming months: as soon as people felt that they themselves were safe, it would be hard to keep them motivated. "It's only people in nursing homes that are at risk" was already becoming a mantra for people arguing for returning to normal. It would be hard for people to understand that they were a link in the chain to the death of someone they didn't know.

Fischhoff made some other essential points. One was that "the human mind is not wired to think about exponential (nonlinear, dynamic) processes. As a result, people need the wisdom to trust the science, not their intuitions." In other words, we are not all my son Zach. Much would turn on how much the public was willing to trust Anthony Fauci and Deborah Birx, the chief scientists on the White House Task Force; if they were undermined, any program was going to fail.

Fischhoff believed that reimposing strict measures after lifting them would be much more challenging, as people react strongly to losing something but are less appreciative of gaining something (like a reduction in restrictions), particularly if they believe they are owed it.

His comments persuaded me that success in controlling the pandemic depended on four factors: leaders who were willing to make unpopular decisions for the good of everyone, human empathy, social cohesion, and a trust in science. In retrospect, we were zero for four, though at the time, in late March, I wasn't so pessimistic. We were in new territory. Besides, we just had to do the best we could.

Fischhoff's perspective also convinced me that talking about things in hyper-local terms was going to be much more effective than throwing out broad statistics. Zach's analysis that each of us can be responsible for 40 lives saved or lost, which I had talked about with Kasie Hunt on MSNBC, was the best way I knew to do that.

Fischhoff forwarded a paper by Harvey Fineberg, the chair of the National Academy of Medicine's Standing Committee on Infectious Diseases. One of the conclusions of the study (which Mike Pence had quietly commissioned) was that the only strategy with strong empirical evidence of effectiveness was the strict Chinese strategy—Bill Joy's view.[24] Fineberg, one of the finest and most credible medical and health policy voices we have in the country, predicted uncontrollable results if social distancing measures were weakened.

The study also said that without strict social distancing, household spread and large numbers of health care workers would keep the disease moving through the population no matter what else we did. *We are embedding failure into the structure of our approach*, I thought.

I learned that Fineberg had sent his document to Pence on March 19. The implication hit me immediately: when Trump announced the Easter Sunday Massacre on March 24, he had already been in possession of a document compiled by the very best, most reputable scientists in the country—and commissioned by the White House, no less—stating unequivocally that putting a lot of people together in a room would be like pouring a gallon of gasoline on a kitchen fire. It was one of the first clues that the United States would not soon see its case count drop to near zero, as usually happened between waves in a pandemic, but would have high levels of new infections continuously.

Why was Trump not getting the message? The sudden visibility of Richard Epstein was a clue. If there was a perfect foil to Harvey Fineberg, it was Epstein. One was the picture of humility and contemplation, chose his words carefully, and offered conclusions backed by impeccable research. The other was well known for his ill-informed ideas and fringe theories. Trump is likely the only president in our history who would have chosen to listen to Epstein over Fineberg.

On March 25, Larry convened a phone call with the team of experts he had assembled to help me come up with guidance to present to Kushner. Most of them believed that introducing any system that allowed states or cities to open fully was destined to fail. Without widespread testing and contact tracing, it was. Others argued against any cooperation with the Trump administration. Several people dismissed the suggestions of others without offering better ideas of their own. There were a few pragmatists, including Fischhoff and people with Homeland Security and risk management backgrounds, but they were drowned out by the naysayers. I left the call with a headache.

Whatever the risks of submitting guidance to Kushner, the risks of not submitting something were higher.

But I still needed details. Lana had been kind enough to sit in on the call and take notes, so I used them to begin a draft of the document for Kushner. We had good ideas, but no agreement on the metrics for when to open the economy or to close it back down if need be. I was irritated and felt like putting the whole thing away, so I did the most helpful thing I could think of—I texted my close friends Jeff and Maria, terrific amateur mixologists, to find out how to make myself an old-fashioned. They filmed a video from their kitchen, and I tried to replicate their work. It was my first ten minutes away from the pandemic in a long time. For about 30 seconds, watching my friends make a craft cocktail in their Alexandria, Virginia, kitchen I had been in so often reminded me of ordinary life and the people I missed.

While I worked on my bartending skills, Lana was slightly more productive: she located New Zealand's excellent color-coded system of gates and conditions for closing and reopening the country. That allowed me to draft a set of metrics for the United States. Then John connected me to Beth Seidenberg, a medical researcher and life sciences investor, who worked with me to validate those metrics.

The heart of the document prepared for Kushner laid out the conditions under which a local community would open or close certain parts of its economy. I suggested we create a national public messaging system to educate Americans about how to stay healthy and safe, and a national real-time intelligence-gathering system to monitor safety levels community by community. The document also included a plan to combine the capacities of government, industry, and the scientific community to generate a research and manufacturing process to turn out antibody tests, treatments, and equipment. At that point, the administration was in a position to ask Congress for whatever support was needed. As with the financial crisis of 2008, if the White House was bold, the public and Congress would be supportive and resources would follow. I encouraged boldness, which would allow people to count on financial support through the length of the pandemic.

I proposed that the level of safety measures needed in each community would be coded red, yellow, or green—red signifying the highest level of restriction and green the lowest—depending on five criteria:

1. Infection rate
2. Availability of testing
3. Availability of PPE
4. Hospital capacity
5. Contact tracing capacity

With these criteria, the skeptics I'd spoken with on the call wouldn't have to worry about the country opening up too quickly—given the sparse availability of tests at that point, no state would be ready to open anytime soon.

I gave the document the most Trumpian title I could muster: "Victory over COVID-19." I repeatedly used phrases like "world's greatest" and "We will be the first country to . . ." Even if his effort was a 4 that could be dressed up as a 6, it would still be better than leading folks to slaughter.

I expected the White House would receive several proposals like this. So I tried to align our main points with the ones likely to appear in other proposals. I also encouraged Kushner to share our paper with others inside and outside the White House so that he could see there was a broad consensus and present that to the president.

On the evening of March 26, I hit send on my message to Kushner and called it a night—by which I mean I checked my texts, did a CNN segment, and got on Twitter.

CHAPTER 5

THE VIRUS AND THE WHITE HOUSE, PART II

SCENE: WASHINGTON STATE AND WASHINGTON, D.C.

Blythe Adamson had just stepped off the plane in Seattle when she felt her phone buzz. It was March 18, and she and her two daughters had decided to leave their New York apartment and ride out the pandemic at the Pacific Northwest oyster farm where she'd grown up. They had been through a lot, having survived domestic violence and living on the edge of homelessness. It would do the girls good to spend time with their grandparents and experience the peace of a remote beach. Adamson herself was looking forward to writing equations near the bald eagles while breathing in the salty smell of the bay.

As they walked to get their bags, she read the text on her phone. It was from Nat Turner, her boss at Flatiron Health, a niche health care company that analyzed data on how to best treat cancer patients. Could she come to the White House as soon as possible? She looked down at Penelope and Daphne, who were peering at the carousel where their bags would soon arrive. Several years ago, her family had been relying on food stamps. Though they were now thriving, it was hard to escape the feeling that it might not last. Adamson woke up many nights worried about keeping her children safe and putting enough food on the table.

Could she go to the White House? Adamson was not a Republican and tried hard to stay out of politics. Numbers were her thing. She was an academic scientist trained as both an economist and an infectious disease epidemiologist—one of only a small number in the country. She had spent the last few years developing models for how to best care for cancer patients. Turner had given her the freedom to build the most sophisticated analytical capabilities in the world. Working with the most complex health data, she coded in six languages and spun models out of her brain. She could speak both health and economics fluently: trade-offs, dynamic assumptions, deep analytics.

No, she decided, going to D.C. would be impossible. The girls needed her; never mind what she thought about the man in the Oval Office. She would have to say she was flattered, but obviously this was out of the question. She dialed Turner's number and leaned against the wall as she talked to him, trying to understand the gravity of the situation, while Penelope and Daphne made big plans to build a clubhouse in the woods.

After the long drive out to Puget Sound, the next day she was back at the airport and headed for the White House. But first she needed to stop by her apartment in New York, since all she had packed to shelter in place was sweatpants.

Fighting COVID-19 with Weapons for the Flu

By the time Adamson arrived the following day at a makeshift bullpen at FEMA, Jared Kushner was frustrated. That agency, along with HHS and the White House, needed to make a series of decisions to secure and distribute supplies, but they had very little evidence to inform those decisions. The White House wouldn't publicly acknowledge the CDC testing error, but without tests they had almost no way to estimate what was going to happen. Kushner had questions, most of which he thought it should be simple to answer, such as: How many ventilators were going to be needed at the peak of the pandemic? How about gowns, gloves, and masks? Was it as bad as the Democratic governors were making it out to be? The answers were supposed to be coming from teams at the CDC and HHS, which had been tasked with creating a model for how the virus would spread. But they were not providing any answers. They needed a first-class model, the kind few people could create quickly.

Adamson assessed the situation. The mathematicians at the CDC and at the division of HHS known as the Office of the Assistant Secretary for Preparedness and Response (ASPR) had in fact been working tirelessly for weeks to model the spread of the coronavirus, but they were having trouble. In one of her first conversations, she discovered the problem: they had taken a shortcut that resulted in a substantial error. They were basing their model on a previous model they had developed—but it was a model used to project the spread of influenza, not COVID-19, and flu and COVID-19 are transmitted very differently. Flu spreads only when the carrier has symptoms, by which time people generally stay home, whereas COVID-19 can spread when the carrier has no symptoms. Throwing COVID-19 cases into a model of flu transmission gave the mathematicians much lower infection numbers than the coronavirus was actually producing.

This put the alphabet soup of government agencies in a pickle. Not only were their model numbers not matching what the country was experiencing, but the CDC and ASPR teams were unwilling to share the details of their models, inputs, assumptions, or programming code with FEMA, the White House's task force, the Office of Science and Technology Policy (OSTP), or the Council of Economic Advisors (CEA).

Adamson recognized that the mathematicians were doing the best they could with the tools they had. Legitimate dynamic transmission models—models that allow you to simulate what happens as variables such as human behavior change—normally take years to build, and once you have them, it takes days to run each simulation. Even the CDC's flu-based model required 19 hours to run a single simulation. Adamson knew that even if a model could spit out the right answer, it would need to run fast or else it would never be used.

Speed of information is everything in a crisis. During the Healthcare.gov turnaround, it was only when we could see exactly where people were getting tripped up on the website in real time that we knew what to fix. And before we fixed something, we had to understand how that would affect people's experience elsewhere on the website. Now, though, it was late March and the White House did not have basic visibility into the impact of the virus or the specific demands that would fall on the health care system. This would be like fighting a fire without knowing where it is, how big it is, and how much tinder there is near it.

That's why Adamson was here.

Soon after she arrived in D.C., an armored black government SUV came to pick her up at FEMA headquarters and take her to the White House. After a long walk from where the SUV dropped her, she went through a guard station, then a temperature-checking station, and then another guard station with metal detectors before entering the side door on the lower level of the West Wing.

After walking up one flight of steps, she entered the Roosevelt Room, a nicely decorated all-purpose conference room with photographs of both Theodore Roosevelt and Franklin Delano Roosevelt. Opposite from the door she entered was a door leading to White House staff offices and another right outside the Oval Office from which the president enters the room. Couches and chairs line the walls behind the conference table. The custom is for principals and important guests to sit at the table, with staff lining the back wall. One chair at the table was different from all the others, with a slightly higher back; if the president wasn't in the room, whoever ran the meeting could sit in it.

Adamson took a seat against the back wall. Gathered in the room were Deborah Birx, the economic team, and a team from

OSTP. Birx was at the end of the table, leading the meeting. In front of Adamson at the table was a skinny guy whose job seemed to be to make sure Birx had everything she needed to do her work; Adamson thought this man must be Birx's chief of staff.

Deborah Birx was raised on a farm in Amish country in Pennsylvania.[1] Her father was a mathematician, and she grew up with a love of science. She finished college in two years, got her medical degree at Penn State, and joined the army, where she became a colonel. She worked as a physician at Walter Reed Medical Center and did HIV research at a laboratory under Anthony Fauci in the NIH. She served in the CDC and then as the United States global AIDS coordinator under Barack Obama before being appointed by Vice President Pence as the coordinator for the White House Coronavirus Task Force. In her early sixties, Birx was composed, poised, and whip-smart, with an occasionally sharp temper. She was held in high regard by the scientific community, and with her background in infectious disease, she was well suited for the work of this task force.

She, too, craved numbers. In the meeting, Birx pleaded for more information from the CDC, putting Robert Redfield, the CDC director, in the hot seat. He said the CDC was working on getting its model together but that it wasn't ready to be presented. Birx seemed understanding but frustrated. Adamson was practically jumping out of her skin because she knew what needed to be done, but she stayed quiet.

Afterward she talked to the CDC team. The last thing she wanted to do was undermine them. She agreed to start building a model that could be used by Birx, Kushner, and the economic team as a bridge, while assisting the CDC modelers in finalizing their work. On March 20, the day after she arrived, she had a model up and running.

At a subsequent meeting, when it came out that the CDC analysis still was not yet finished, the skinny guy became even more frustrated. "What do you want to do? Write a history book?" he asked the CDC team. By that time, Adamson had identified the impatient skinny guy not as Birx's chief of staff but as Jared Kushner.

What Adamson saw from her perch was chaos—more than

your standard fog-of-war chaos, where facts are coming in fast. The National Economic Council (NEC) argued for reopening the economy, while Birx and Fauci disagreed strenuously, but without a single set of data or a reliable model, neither side had the numbers to support their argument. As absurd as NEC chair Larry Kudlow's public comment about our control of the virus being "airtight" was, there was nothing to refute it. Where we actually stood was anybody's guess. Trump had finally acknowledged the pandemic, but the White House Task Force working on it was stuck.

It wasn't only Politics with a capital P, the politics of elections and perceptions, but politics with a lower-case p, the politics of who has power, gets credit, or looks good to the boss, that hampered the White House and the country.

Sunny Optimism in the West Wing

At the end of March, I was appearing on TV and writing on Twitter and in national publications, trying to prepare the country for what I believed would be one of the most deadly months in U.S. history. With Adamson's help and cases leveling off, Birx appeared to be enjoying her newfound status, having daily chats in the Oval Office with the president and Kushner. In a White House news conference, she showed slides of how things were getting better every day. Now that we were beginning to stay home, she believed, we were on track to follow the path of Italy, which had rapidly improved. Her pronouncements reflected Trump's sunny optimism, and in turn, the promise of good news buoyed the president and Kushner. The pandemic would soon be behind them, they thought; the United States was entering the comeback phase Kushner had predicted. Little did Birx know that the White House was about to begin abdicating responsibility for battling the virus.

Because she understood how both the scientists and the economic team worked, Adamson had been able to develop a working model that all the teams could use. She even incorporated data indicating how much less Americans were moving around. The economic team trusted her model and used it to simulate various scenarios. And her work could serve as a bridge that gave the CDC time to finish up its efforts to create a more detailed model of disease spread. She collaborated with people she thought were doing excellent work, including the CEA team; Admiral Brett Giroir, the assistant secretary for health at HHS; and Colonel Pat Work, a key army leader at FEMA. She was quickly becoming a star. She even had a small office on the lower level of the West Wing. The one thing she refused to do was own any of the assumptions. The purpose of transparent modeling, she believed, was to allow the various teams to arrive at a consensus.

On March 26, with the CDC still not having produced its own model, Kushner began to take interest in a model developed by the Institute for Health Metrics and Evaluation (IHME), an independent population health research center at the University of Washington. It was the first academic institution in the United States willing to put a stake in the ground. An Imperial College London model released on March 16 had estimated that the death toll in the United States would be between 1 million and 2 million. The IHME model had a very different estimate, one Kushner and the president liked a lot better: 60,000 total deaths.[2] The team who checked it out, including Birx, said it was credible. The fact that two recognized institutions could put out two vastly different projections was itself a sign of how little was known.

On March 28, Trump felt there was a light at the end of the tunnel. There had been fewer than 3,000 deaths thus far. While Fauci was warning that up to 200,000 Americans could die if things weren't handled well, Birx was telling the president that the death rate would peak in two weeks and then begin to drop as Americans sustained their new habits of staying home and social distancing. Compared to 2 million deaths, 60,000 felt like a home run. Seeing the end in sight, Trump encouraged Americans to follow social distancing guidelines until April 30.

John Doerr called when he saw the news.

"Hey, we won one!" John said into the phone, relieved that Trump was no longer insisting that the country open up by Easter Sunday.

"Yes. Thank God," I replied, and mentioned that I'd heard it from Kushner, who'd said our "Victory over COVID-19" paper had helped make the case.

"Jared read the paper?" he asked.

"He said he had. It sounds like they will use some of it in their approach to opening up."

"When do you think that will be?"

"In a perfect world, it would be June—there aren't nearly enough tests to even know where the outbreaks are or how quickly things are growing. But Trump said the end of April. I doubt he will extend it. We need a dramatic drop in cases before then, and we have to push states to go slow and follow the plan," I said. "If not, all we did was buy a few weeks."

On March 31, Adamson was packing up and getting ready to return to the West Coast to reunite with her girls. Leaving the White House with a model they could use until the CDC model was complete meant that her job was done. As she walked through the West Wing, she bumped into Kushner, who had just come from an optimistic meeting at which Birx shared her confidence that cases were continuing to decline. Kushner said to Adamson with a grin, "If things go well, we may be able to open even sooner."

We're not there yet, she thought. She decided her job wasn't done, so she called Turner at Flatiron and told him she needed to stay a while longer.

The IHME model the White House was relying on was deeply flawed. In early April, I participated in a Zoom call with Chris Murray, the principal modeler from IHME, who was sharing the contents of the model the White House was using and explaining the assumptions behind his estimate capping the U.S. death toll at only 60,000. Murray's model assumed a few things that were highly implausible: that states wouldn't have any more outbreaks, that social distancing standards wouldn't be relaxed, that there would be no interstate or international travel, and that the transmission rate would drop below 1.0 (meaning the average infected person would infect fewer than one other person) and remain there. He also assumed that no state would open up if it had more than 10 cases.[3] These inputs did not pass the common sense test. Immediately after hearing them, I published those clearly flawed assumptions to Twitter. (In early May, Murray revised his estimate upward after it was clear how far off the assumptions were.)[4]

Despite this estimate being so obviously wrong in so many ways, on April 20, backed by Birx, Trump announced to the country that the final death toll of the virus in the United States would be 50,000 to 60,000. He added that his actions had already saved "a million people, maybe two million people."[5] The administration was declaring victory. One person in the White House told me the total deaths would likely cap out at 30,000. Birx publicly attributed the great results to the president and lavished praise on him in meetings and, more importantly, on camera.

A former Democratic senator called and asked me if I thought Birx had gone over to the "dark side."

I was more forgiving of her comments. "She's working the judge," I said. "But her optimism isn't well founded."

My Twitter soon blew up with people gleefully telling me this was proof that I was nothing but a fearmonger for having suggested the death toll could be a lot higher. I made no argument back. I had no interest in accepting more deaths; besides, those epidemiological estimates were not mine to defend. But I worried that these fantastical IHME estimates would render short-lived any gains we had been able to make by pushing state reopenings beyond Easter.

But Trump's White House was a marketing machine, not a problem-solving machine.

"If we did this a different way, we would have lost more—much more than 2 million people. And we did it the right way. We did everything right," Trump said, taking credit for the difference between the IHME projection and the Imperial College London projection.[6]

It was no surprise that Trump misused both estimates, but Birx's support was another matter. With the low estimates that Birx supported, the economists from the NEC who were on the task force had essentially prevailed in their debate with the public health people to get the country open more quickly. Michael Shear, the White House correspondent for the *New York Times*, described Birx as an outright cheerleader for opening up the country.[7] Was she influenced by trying to please the president, or did she just miss something basic?

I had a chance to talk to her about this when I met with her in person in August in Minnesota. She told me that she'd been so impressed with the public's response to social distancing in early April that she'd assumed it would be sustained until June, by which time she thought states could safely open up. She saw what had happened in Italy as that country recovered, and thought the United States would do the same. If she had spent five minutes with Baruch Fischhoff trying to understand human motivation instead of inhaling the groupthink of the White House, I think she would have had a different perspective. What she failed to grasp was all the ways the United States was not like Italy. Like a lot of places in the world, Italy was hit with a second wave, but in the meantime, it had saved a lot of lives by reducing the case count and death toll; its number of deaths per capita was one-quarter that of the United States' number. But the differences between Italy and the United States—different leaders, different cultures, different views of science, different ability to commit to collective action—are what much of this book is about. She didn't account for the fact that the United States stood alone in devolving responsibility away from the federal government. By the time I saw her in August, her early optimism was long gone.

What was also clear was that we didn't have the kind of leadership in the White House that asked tough questions or acknowledged bad news. Trump had already demonstrated that when Azar presented him with dire warnings. And the task force that was in place, led by an acquiescent Pence, wasn't going to change that approach. If Trump wanted to open up the country by Easter, he had found his team. If he wanted to affirm to the stock market that things weren't going to be very bad, he had found his team. Unfortunately for him and us, pandemics don't respond to wishful thinking.

Choosing Politics over Health and the Economy

In the very long days and nights during the Healthcare.gov turn-around in 2013, my job was simple: getting insurance to anyone who wanted it. That one goal carried the day in every decision I made. When Tim Geithner was leading the country out of the financial crisis as treasury secretary, the most important thing was restoring economic stability. When you're driven by a clear goal, hard choices such as bailing out the banks are easier to make. If you are to have any hope of managing a big crisis successfully, you must decide what the single most important thing is and simply do the best you can with everything else. The bigger and more complex the challenge is, the more important that rule is. And for a country under attack the way the United States was from COVID-19, *saving the next life* would appear to a reasonable person to be the single most important objective. (Indeed, when I joined the Biden White House with the crisis still raging as of Inauguration Day, I taped that statement to my desk and was driven by it every day.)

Trump and others have frequently said we shouldn't "make the cure worse than the problem itself." Whenever he mentioned this, the examples he cited most frequently were mental health issues, a slump in the economy, and children missing school.[8] While, as I said earlier, the evidence is that the pandemic, not the response, is the main culprit for the negative effects in those areas, there is a legitimate point here about doing the best job possible addressing those issues. Trump, however, didn't propose an additional dollar in spending for mental health, for retrofitting schools, or for adding broadband, and after a time, he even lost interest in supporting the small businesses hurt by the pandemic.

So what was Trump's priority? The economy? The stock market? Those things were clearly important to him, but when push came to shove, even those goals were less important than one thing—*avoiding accountability.*

Even back at the end of March, when the administration was warning of as many as 240,000 deaths, Trump's guiding principle was to blame someone else. Blue states (where the initial outbreaks were centered), Congress, China, the CDC, and the FDA were all handy spots to place blame, not only for those losses but for any challenges citizens were facing because of the pandemic.

By April, there were the first signs that the growth in the number of new pandemic cases was finally beginning to slow. The #StayHome efforts of Americans, buoyed by states' stay-at-home orders and Trump's reluctant support, were finally beginning to reduce case counts.

As I sat in my breakfast nook having coffee with Lana one morning in early April, Jared Kushner's name again flashed on my phone. I picked up, and he was polite and appreciative of my past help. He told me he felt like we were getting to a good place. I imagine he meant that at least things were feeling less chaotic and some of the immediate fires, like that of finding enough ventilators, had been snuffed out. We caught up on a few topics, and I pushed for an increase in testing, as I had in our last couple of calls. It seemed obvious that there was no way to meet any of the reopening criteria without more testing, and the federal government needed to help.

"We're going to put testing back to the states," Kushner said. "We can't be responsible. We've given them everything they need, but they won't solve this unless we make them own it. Some of them clearly don't want to succeed. Bad incentives to keep blaming us."

What he described was more of a political strategy than a public health strategy. Trump would announce that the country would be reopening at the end of the month, but states would have to solve the hard problems. This way, if things opened and went badly, Trump could point to the governors. If there weren't enough diagnostic tests, the states could be blamed. The implication was stunning but not entirely surprising. Governors were going to get abandoned. Many states wouldn't have enough tests for months. The combination of opening by the end of the month, a lack of tests, and the White House's efforts to avoid blame seemed like a surefire way for cases to grow.

I had talked to several governors over the last several days. All they wanted was more forceful White House support. I felt like the president and his team were surrendering the war.

"No, Jared. I don't think that's true. The states need a partnership," I countered.

Kushner said their minds were made up.

I tried again. If the White House didn't maintain responsibility, I said, cases would grow and the states would be helpless without the support of the federal government. But Kushner wouldn't budge.

The import was clear to me: they were abdicating responsibility.

To Boldly Go Where No Man Has Gone Before

Peter Marks was a *Star Trek* fan from Brooklyn. He's a physician with a PhD in cell and molecular biology. After a career in academic medicine and·a stint in the pharmaceutical industry, Marks found his calling—as a regulator. Marks is the man at the FDA in charge of approving vaccines and other innovative therapies. On the morning of April 7, while the White House was beginning to figure out how to extract themselves from the pandemic response, Marks was figuring out how to go in deeper. A career civil servant, he wasn't paying attention to the political jockeying in the administration; he wanted to collapse a multiyear vaccine evaluation process into months and had an idea of how to do it. He picked up the phone and called Rick Bright at the Biomedical Advanced Research and Development Authority (BARDA), one of the men who had been instrumental in BARDA's investment in new vaccine technologies.

Together with Anthony Fauci, whose team had worked with the pioneers of this new vaccine technology called messenger-RNA (or mRNA), they had access to the best expertise and infrastructure for conducting clinical trials, they came up with a plan that Marks dubbed "Operation Warp Speed." The plan would call for assigning specific teams from the NIH, BARDA, and the FDA to work hand in hand with five or six of the most promising vaccine developers and minimize the back-and-forth customary in the drug approval process. Bright believed that with the right financial support, the government could fund vaccine manufacturing even while the trials were ongoing. It was a risky financial bet, but if it worked, it would accelerate a vaccine by six months. Between Marks, Fauci, and Bright, they believed they had a chance to get a vaccine to the public inside of a year.

At that point, none of Trump's political appointees were aware of the plan. So on April 10, the scientists presented it to the HHS secretary. To this point, Azar had been concerned vaccines would take too long, and so he had been focused instead on therapies to minimize the virus's effects. When he heard the plan the scientists presented, he liked it and signed off on it.

The Final Nail

Leading up to Birx's announcement in mid-April, Kushner walked into the office of Trump's new chief of staff, Mark Meadows, to discuss what he had told me about: the state authority handoff. The president would announce the new opening strategy and from there leave it to the states to implement. It seemed to be a clever political strategy, because it would help Trump avoid taking continued blame from blue-state governors and begin to shift the blame to them. If there was a high death toll or if there was insufficient testing, it wouldn't be on the Trump administration.

On the afternoon of April 16, Trump had a phone call with governors in which he told them, "You are going to call your own shots."[9] In the evening, Birx led a White House press briefing in which she rolled out the White House opening guidelines for states;

they were very close to what we had submitted in the "Victory over COVID-19" plan. She announced that the distancing recommendations the federal government had put in place would disappear on April 30.[10] These guidelines would be used in their place.

Shortly after the White House foisted responsibility for the pandemic onto states, Adam Boehler was reassigned to his old duties overseeing international investments at the U.S. International Development Finance Corporation, and the White House sidelined the task force and ended the regular briefings to the nation.

Every few weeks we could delay the country's reopening gave scientists more time to discover better treatments and gave doctors and nurses a chance for a breather. But despite buying time between Easter Sunday and the end of the month, I had mixed feelings about contributing to the White House plan. As I noted in Chapter 3, in the United States, like in other nations, only the federal government was positioned to oversee a coherent strategy to respond to the pandemic in close partnership with local officials. Only the federal government could adequately access the funding, the research, and the resources. Without its oversight, the states would be forced into bidding wars for those resources.

Two days after the April 16 state authority handoff announcement, Kushner discussed it in an interview with Bob Woodward that wasn't made public until October.[11] He said issuing the guidelines "was almost like Trump getting the country back from the doctors." And his spin on the federal government abdicating its role in managing the pandemic was that "the states have to own the testing. The federal government should not own the testing. . . . But the president also is very smart politically with the way he did that fight with the governors to basically say, no, no, no, no, I own the opening. Because again, the opening is going to be very popular. People want this country open. But if it opens in the wrong way, the question will be, did the governors follow the guidelines we set out or not?"

I had once heard Obama use a basketball expression along the lines of "Some people like to have the ball in their hands in the fourth quarter and some people don't." Trump wanted no part of the ball. To me, this was responsibility avoidance, dressed up in clever politics—and leading to death.

This approach was also far from the stroke of political genius Kushner was describing. He was mistaken if he thought the White House could avoid responsibility if the death toll continued to rise, as the decision to reopen at the end of April seemed to guarantee. As the country headed toward the November presidential election, the politics never moved in Trump's direction. COVID-19 did become a top election issue, but not in a way that favored Trump.

Despite the scientists advising against it, by the end of April states began to open up. And history shows the consequences of what followed. As the Pulitzer Prize–winning journalist Connie Schultz later said to me, you can fix a lot of things, but "you can't un-die people."

CHAPTER 6

TRUMP EATS THE MARSHMALLOW

Scene: The political arena

"Mr. President, do you mind if I tell you a bedtime story?"

Having extended her stay in Washington, Blythe Adamson was playing a pivotal role with the scientific and economic teams in the White House as a go-to source for analysis of what might come next with the pandemic.

Her first meeting with Trump took place on April 6. It was set up as a quick Oval Office photo op to thank her and the other volunteers, but when the president invited them all to stay, it turned into a 45-minute bull session. Trump loved showing off the Oval Office, much more than Obama, who had been stingier about using it as a showplace.

Each of the volunteers introduced themselves briefly to the president. All were men except Adamson, and to her they all seemed like Ivy Leaguers, well off and confident, the kind of men she had gotten used to seeing all around New York. They used their introductions to highlight their personal achievements. Trump was impressed with people who had made a lot of money. If someone had sold a company, he wanted to know how much they sold it for.

What would the president and all the rest of them think, Adamson wondered, if they knew she used to live on public assistance? Or that she had escaped domestic violence? When her turn came, she introduced herself as an economist and an epidemiologist.

Upon hearing her credentials, Trump clearly wanted to engage with her. "So, you believe the Chinese made this virus in a lab, right?" he said to her.

Adamson paused. How should she answer this? She had studied zoonotic viruses—viruses that spill over to humans from other animals—for years, and she knew it was extremely unlikely that this virus had been engineered in a lab. Agreeing with his statement was out of the question, but disagreeing with the president seemed like a delicate matter.

So she asked if she could tell the president a bedtime story. The dozen men in the room glanced at each other and grew very still and silent.

Trump was impressed by her confidence. How could he say no?

"There was a beautiful tropical jungle in Africa," she began, "with wildflowers and animals. People in villages would always have to walk around the jungle because it was too hard to get through. Because of the hassle that came from traveling around the jungle, they decided to tear it down to build a road. The workers building this road did not have time to stop and build fires for cooking food and so instead would eat bushmeat—raw or minimally processed meat—from monkeys that inhabited the jungle."

Here she looked at her main audience. He was leaning forward without blinking.

"What the workers did not know, however, was that a virus was present in the monkeys they were eating. Very quickly, a worker got sick from the virus and passed it on to other humans."

She paused again, meeting the president's gaze. He wasn't used to someone controlling the conversation quite the way Adamson had and was hanging on her every word.

"And that's the story of HIV."

"Really?" Trump asked, eyes wide with astonishment.

"There are lots of viruses that live in animals without hurting them. The moral of the story is that when we do something to mess up nature, that makes viruses spill over into humans. It's way more likely that this coronavirus is a random spillover from animals to humans than that it was engineered by someone in a lab in China."

Researchers are still studying precisely how humans were infected with SARS-CoV-2, the coronavirus that causes COVID-19. As with the genetically similar SARS virus, which generated a global outbreak in 2002–2003, the clues suggested a jump from animals to humans.[1] The more humans expand into the habitats of wild animals, the more likely these viruses are to make their way to humans.

As Ed Yong wrote in a 2016 article in *The Atlantic* titled "How a Pandemic Might Play Out Under Trump": "By encroaching into the territories of wild animals, we provide the sparks for new pandemics. By living in increasingly crowded urban areas, we provide the tinder."[2]

Just One Marshmallow

There's a famous 1972 experiment in which researchers put a small child in a room with a marshmallow and offer a choice. The child can eat the marshmallow or, if they wait 15 minutes without eating the marshmallow, they receive a second one. That study linked the ability to delay gratification with better educational and other outcomes.[3] But sometimes patience and discipline don't come easy.

To understand the state authority handoff is to understand one of the biggest miscalculations in the entire COVID-19 response. It is best approached by looking at some of the peculiarities of President Trump's decision-making process and how his staff briefs him on important options. Trump understood relatively little about how the government operated compared to the people responsible for briefing him, so it was easy for the staff to provide only options they wanted him to consider. In 2017, Zeke Emanuel witnessed this when he met with Trump and his team to try to convince them not to press forward with repealing the ACA. In the meeting, then–

House Speaker Paul Ryan and then–chief of staff Reince Priebus told Trump that he had only two options for repealing the ACA and that he had to choose one of them or else he wouldn't be able to get a large tax cut passed. To which Zeke characteristically replied, "With all due respect, that's not true. You're the president of the United States. You have practically unlimited options." Of course, the ACA wasn't repealed, and Trump got his tax cut anyway.

Trump needed to be treated like he was the smartest person in the room, and if he already had a point of view, dissent was generally unwelcome (bedtime stories possibly excluded). If you knew what it was he wanted, briefings were best focused on how to give it to him, not on changing his mind. By the time the pandemic hit, his staff was mostly down to Trump-pleasers—people who wouldn't risk angering him with a challenging recommendation.

All of this makes it possible to understand one simple but still amazing point: in March and April, no one had presented Trump with an option that would have saved the greatest number of lives—a national plan for controlling the pandemic consistent with what countries all over the globe were successfully doing. This option was not presented because it was expressly understood to be something Trump wouldn't consider. In fact, despite the availability of Adamson's model, which allowed any number of scenarios to be looked at, it wasn't even considered worthwhile for the team to analyze options they knew Trump wouldn't favor; this included any extended restrictions on the economy or anything that kept responsibility with the federal government.

Across the globe, countries were significantly reducing the spread of the coronavirus by implementing a series of measures around which there was a growing consensus: a national mask mandate, rapid testing, temporary isolation of those with the virus, mandatory quarantines after foreign travel, and closing down crowded indoor places where the virus most easily spreads. Whether countries had been prepared initially, as South Korea was, or taken by surprise, as Italy was, these actions were quickly containing the virus.

When a second wave of cases hit Europe in the fall of 2020,

countries rolled out the exact same set of measures and again achieved the same result. Dealing with an outbreak that starts from a minimal number of cases and a more rested public is like fighting a rabid dog; fighting multiple outbreaks from a high initial case count is like fighting packs of rabid dogs.

If the United States had taken a similar set of actions, we would likely have gotten the country back to a near-normal state in six weeks, with only small handfuls of cases.[4] I wrote an editorial in *USA Today* and did a media tour to discuss the approach. My message was simple: We are always six to eight weeks from crushing the virus (at least for an extended period) anytime we choose. However, that would have required discipline, clear communication, and no small measure of sacrifice. And because it was so challenging, it would also have required leadership. Such a difficult task would have had the greatest chance of success in spring and summer of 2020, when the public was not yet suffering from pandemic fatigue. And it would have had the benefit of creating a rising economy and a safe public environment before the school year started (and the election season began). Most important, untold numbers of lives would have been saved.

Despite the near-uniform success of this approach in other countries, it was understood that the president would not consider it, so no one at the White House analyzed it, let alone presented it to him. Instead, Deborah Birx offered a plan for success without federal involvement—while still assuming all of the benefits these other countries had achieved. Birx didn't consider that states might choose to treat the guidelines as optional—and certainly not that they would ignore them almost entirely. Her focus instead was on convincing Trump to support her plan. She played to his penchant for public flattery. "He's been so attentive to the scientific literature and the details and the data," she said in a TV interview in late March. "I think his ability to analyze and integrate data that comes out of his long history in business has really been a real benefit during these discussions about medical issues."[5]

Birx believed things were improving, as she saw the benefit of

Americans staying at home, including data Adamson provided her that people were moving around their communities less. But Birx's and Fauci's approaches stood in contrast. She expressed optimism; he expressed caution. Fauci described himself as the "skunk at the garden party" and cautioned against all the happy talk, reminding people that "models are only models"; how accurate they would be depended on how successfully people adhered to restrictions on their behavior.[6]

Birx confidently presented the "Opening Up America Again" guidelines at an April 16 press conference with the president.[7] But it was soon clear that she and the president had two different interpretations of what they were doing. To Birx, this was the road map back. To the president, this was the state authority handoff, the moment when he would, to use Kushner's words, start "getting the country back from the doctors."

Less than 24 hours later, Trump's intentions became obvious. Small groups of protesters and Trump supporters showed up outside the residence of Minnesota governor Tim Walz, a Democrat, to protest the ongoing public health restrictions—the very restrictions outlined in Birx's reopening guidelines, which Trump had endorsed the day before. Men with firearms also entered the state capitol in the battleground state of Michigan to protest against Democratic governor Gretchen Whitmer for the same reason. And then the president tweeted, "LIBERATE MICHIGAN!" and "LIBERATE MINNESOTA!"[8]

Trump had devoured the marshmallow in one bite. Any hope of a successful response was gone.

Dave Calouri, one of the volunteers on the White House team, saw Trump's tweets. He walked over to Adamson's desk in the basement of the West Wing and asked if she had seen them. She hadn't; she didn't pay much attention to politics or presidential tweets. He filled her in on the tweets and then on the situations in Minnesota and Michigan.

"Can you check and see if these states are ready to open based on the criteria we laid out yesterday?" he asked.

Adamson did a quick analysis, then shook her head. "They're not. What should I do with that?"

"Call the lawyers and tell them," Dave told her.

What Trump had done was more than a populist kick in the shins. He was signaling—not just to a small group in Michigan or Minnesota but to supporters around the country—that, like him, people could rebel against the government's experts. Sometimes when it was required of him, he would grudgingly say what the experts wanted him to, but he would be sure to wink to his followers to show them how he really felt.

If Trump had looked ahead and thought strategically about something he wanted—for example, to open the economy and schools safely and in time for the election—he would have followed Birx's plan while putting into place a national infrastructure of widespread and rapid testing. Instead he ended public focus on the pandemic even as case counts grew again, and tried to will the country to move on to other things. When the fall came, there would be no second marshmallow.

If Birx felt undermined by the president, she knew better than to say anything. Birx later told me that having a president so quickly contradict you happens to everyone. It doesn't, and she knew it.

Trump's Politics of Denial

It's really hard for a leader to do a brilliant, superb job [in a pandemic]. It's really hard to earn an A, but it's super easy to earn a B. . . . To do a good enough job is not so hard. We have seen people who are not extraordinarily capable politicians who understood what you have to do. . . . I think President Trump is just not able to give a coherent explanation of his actions and he's not able to even pretend to perform empathy.

—David Frum on *In the Bubble*, May 2020[9]

"Did you like what we put out tonight??" Jared Kushner texted me after the April 16 press conference (but before Trump's "liberate" tweets invalidated it). He told me that much of the work we had submitted was in there and was a useful baseline, and he offered his thanks. The truth is, if we had operated according to the White House plan *and* if the federal government had provided oversight and resources, it would have saved a lot of lives.

Trump's denial of the pandemic as it came to our shores was costly. According to a Columbia University report, if we had implemented social distancing and other control measures one week earlier, we would have saved 36,000 lives by May 3.[10] If we'd done it two weeks earlier, we'd have saved 54,000 lives. These were preventable deaths. But it didn't end there. By the time we got to May, and the virus seemed impossible to deny, Trump continued to promise that solutions were coming any day now and that the virus would "just disappear."[11]

Historians will ask why Trump initially chose to deny the existence of the virus and then, when he finally did acknowledge it, kept promising a fix was just around the corner. Setting aside the question of whether he was even bothered by the potential for massive loss of life, might there have been a political advantage to addressing the virus? There is a long history of presidents growing more popular during times of crisis. And certainly no one believed that Trump caused the virus. But he chose instead to mislead the country, to pretend that there was no crisis. Why?

There may be no simpler answer than that it is his nature.

There is a set of personality traits required to face a crisis— particularly when the antagonist is invisible and the public needs to be trained to perceive it: The ability to separate yourself from the problem and continually weigh choices based on current information. The need to focus on the bad news and look skeptically at good news. Empathy for people who aren't right in front of you. A willingness to make tough decisions that forgo short-term gains in favor of solutions that work. The ability to communicate in a way that brings people together. Trump did not possess those traits. He was all gut instinct, with an ego that couldn't accept anything that didn't paint his presidency as an unadulterated success. In his mind, he should have been able to just swat away the coronavirus, say it would magically disappear and make it so.

Trump was from the school where you never show weakness and never admit a mistake. And so the coronavirus persisted and grew exponentially despite his protestations and his efforts to put the responsibility for it on others. If he acknowledged the growing crisis at all, he treated it as an irritant. When the stock market or the polls dipped, he addressed COVID-19 with reluctance and with a throwaway line about how it was going away.

Never could he be made to feel accountable for the mess or people whose lives he could save. Back in April, HHS had planned to mail five reusable face masks to each household in areas with massive infection and rising deaths, places such as New Orleans, Detroit, and New York City.[12] Those 650 million masks would have saved a lot of lives and sent the message that mask wearing was not a political ploy but a safety exercise. The White House killed the idea, as it didn't communicate they were in complete control.

"Insufficient Facts Always Invite Danger"

Operation Warp Speed (OWS) was now being run out of the White House Task Force, and Peter Marks, as its mastermind, was invited to play a leading role. For many, this would have been a plum assignment. It's not every career scientist who gets to brief the vice president in the Situation Room and advise on national strategy. But as his brainchild began to be talked about at press conferences and take on political interest, Marks decided the better place for him was the FDA. The man who developed the vision to accelerate vaccines was soon back at the FDA trying to figure out how to stop his creation from turning into Frankenstein's monster.

The COVID Agendas

Lana is the volunteer elections leader for the Minnesota chapter of the gun-safety group Moms Demand Action. She was an executive at Target headquarters in Minneapolis when she decided that as Cal, our older son, entered middle school, she would shift her energy toward parenting our two boys and local politics. She has been a force of nature in Minnesota political organizing. Many mornings during election season I will wake up to find that she has already been out for hours knocking on doors, or phone banking, or working with a candidate for a local office. While many have urged her to run for office herself, she prefers to be in the background doing the work. Around the house, if something doesn't work, she troubleshoots it, takes it apart, buys replacement parts on the internet, and puts it back together. She's the same way with issues. She reads constantly, remembers virtually everything, and quickly integrates what she has learned into her worldview.

She's about five foot two and scared of no one. If a six-foot-four gun rights supporter with a gun in his belt tries to intimidate her at a protest, she calmly walks right by. One of the things I most frequently hear from people I meet in Minnesota is how much they admire my wife.

When Lana saw the protests in Michigan and Minnesota about ending the temporary shutdown, she saw something I didn't.

"I bet that's the Dorr brothers," she said, and quickly went on the internet to figure it out.

"Who are they? They support gun rights causes?"

"Sort of, but not really."

She explained that the Dorrs were a midwestern family who kept an eye out for conservative causes and would set up nonprofits to raise money off them. Then they would funnel the money into one of their for-profit businesses, including their printing company. The Dorrs weren't ideologues as much as they were opportunists. Conservative organizations launched by the Dorrs have pulled in

$2.9 million just in Iowa, Minnesota, and Ohio since 2013.[13] They quickly seized on the opposition to shutdown measures as another opportunity to stoke the anger of conservative activists—anger that they could leverage to make money for themselves.[14] Within days they had attracted 200,000 people to their anti-lockdown cause by creating Facebook pages called "Minnesotans Against Excessive Quarantine," "Wisconsinites Against Excessive Quarantine," and so on. Each of those pages carried a donation link directing users to the Dorrs' already existing gun rights websites.[15] The president, whether he knew it or not, was supporting the work of these grifters.

I'm pretty sanguine about peaceful protests of any type. Armed protests were another matter. After Michigan survived a major onslaught of COVID-19 cases, I talked to Governor Whitmer on June 15 to get advice we could pass along to the southern governors who were just beginning to see outbreaks in their states.

Whitmer had lost three loved ones to COVID-19 and had recently met with the parents of Skylar Herbert, a five-year-old girl who also died from the disease. She lamented what had become the "politicization of public health."[16] If that politicization wasn't hatched in Michigan, the state was certainly one of the most visible break points from the comity of the early days, when Congress passed big bipartisan relief packages.

Of course, there are protests and then there are protests. Trump was specific about which rebels he supported. After a Minneapolis police officer murdered George Floyd by strangling him slowly with his knee, people mostly wearing masks flooded the streets of the city.[17] In a tweet about the protesters that Twitter flagged as glorifying violence, Trump said, "These THUGS are dishonoring the memory of George Floyd, and I won't let that happen. Just spoke to Governor Tim Walz and told him that the Military is with him all the way. Any difficulty and we will assume control but, when the looting starts, the shooting starts."[18] Governor Walz reported to me that Trump had told him he should "just shoot them."

The erosion of the bipartisan veneer continued little by little. When I did congressional briefings or hearings in March and early April, Democrats and Republicans asked similar questions, focused on how they could prevent loss of life and solve problems in their regions. By late April and May, I began to notice a change. I took sharp questioning from Republicans about how overhyped the virus was and heard much more skepticism about Congress making financial commitments to improve public health. In an email to Andrew Schwab, a United States of Care staffer who was working on crafting legislation to address the crisis, one prominent senator's chief of staff referred to "being held up by the public health mafia." The common line of questioning made it clear that Trump's talking points had been circulated around the congressional offices.

There is often a silver lining to difficult times, whether it be a war or a pandemic. Politics are set aside as we pull together to face a common threat. We'd seen it in the aftermath of 9/11. That's not what was happening in 2020, though. And our division gave aid and comfort to our enemy, the virus.

To make matters worse, proxy political wars developed as a show of support for Trump. When Trump touted hydroxychloroquine as an effective drug despite no proof that it worked and evidence of risk of harm, where you stood on that issue became a matter of political identity.[19] The investment banking firm Goldman Sachs, the Federal Reserve, and the management consulting company McKinsey issued studies demonstrating that masks would reduce transmission of the virus and improve the economy.[20] Nonetheless, when the president decided he would not wear a mask, it became a political statement whether to wear or not wear one.[21] Campaign events at both the federal and state levels were often predominantly maskless if the candidate was Republican, masked if Democratic, from the candidate down to most attendees. New York and San Francisco became mask-wearing cities, joining major urban centers such as Hong Kong and Singapore, which had suffered prior viral outbreaks.[22] Many elected officials and citizens in Georgia, Texas,

Arizona, and Florida, and in rural parts of most states, on the other hand, largely resisted mask wearing on principle, and circulation of the virus accelerated there.[23]

As the death toll increased, many Trump supporters were hard-pressed to even acknowledge it. Often they blamed the increased number of deaths on other diseases, or accused hospitals of lying about patients' cause of death for financial reasons.[24] By the same token, I found Trump's opponents were sometimes too reluctant to acknowledge good news when it happened, such as the reduction in death rates that resulted from improved treatment protocols. Some of Trump's opponents also didn't adequately acknowledge or discuss the challenges of the stay-at-home orders, which included increases in mental illness and domestic abuse, pressures faced by small businesses, and those who lost their lives to other causes because they couldn't access medical care.[25]

Soon reactions turned reflexive. When Democrats expressed horror at the loss of life, Republicans cried election-year politicking.[26] Item after item became a political controversy. In-person schooling, football season, church services, bars and restaurants, progress on a vaccine—all of these became brand-new litmus tests to show which side you were on.

Public health officials even began to receive death threats for calling for masks.[27] In October, a group of extremists was arrested as they plotted to kidnap Governor Whitmer and hold an extrajudicial trial for treason.[28] In some cases families and friends were no longer on speaking terms—not always because of their politics, but because of how they chose to approach the virus. You could feel the patience of the country wearing thin.

In advance of a podcast episode I did titled "How to Talk to Each Other About Wearing Masks," I sent a tweet out one night asking people to call or email if they had a situation with friends, co-workers, or families they wanted to ask about. When I checked in the morning, I found that calls had come in at a rate of two per minute the entire night.[29]

The cost of Trump's political games was high. He poured fuel on a fire he should have been controlling. He took what would have been natural exhaustion and helped it become a cultural war cry. I thought of Bill Joy's analysis that 100,000 lives would be lost for each 10 percent of the public that didn't follow basic public health guidance like mask wearing, and I wondered how much more the president was adding to the death toll every day.

CHAPTER 7

NO ONE LEFT IN CHARGE BUT THE VIRUS

SCENE: EAST, SOUTH, WEST, AND NORTH

We had a crisis at home, and it involved toilet paper. Not that we didn't have any; we were among the lucky families who did. It was that somebody was eating it all . . . along with the spare napkins and surgical masks. Our dog seemed to prefer paper to food. And if one of us caught him with a wad of paper in his mouth, Brodie looked right at us and dared us to come and get it.

It was chaos all over the country, and the Edina war room was no exception. Brodie had a paper mask he had snatched from the counter between his teeth and was running clockwise through the rooms of the house. I finally gave up and called John Doerr to talk through with him my conversation with Kushner and the federal government's abdication of pandemic leadership. When he heard the details, he was despondent. We had averted two potential disasters— the first in March, when people began to stay home, and the second in April, when we avoided the Easter Sunday Massacre—but now we were at an impasse. As we moved through April, the country, abandoned by the Trump administration, seemed to be out of gas for May. I remembered Bill Joy telling me not to enable Trump by sending him a plan that would allow him to shirk responsibility. I had told myself, *We're saving the next life, and besides, what else can we do?* But I was concerned. We had developed criteria for opening up the country, but with the White House having used them to get itself off the hook, they were now being ignored. I feared chaos and wondered whether we'd done the right thing.

"What should we do at this point?" John, as always, was focused on where we were, not how we'd gotten here.

"Focus on the states."

But John reminded me of the obvious: "I'm really worried. That's not nearly as good."

He was right. How was our model of federalism supposed to work in this pandemic? I thought about each state's borders with others—Kentucky with Tennessee, Wisconsin connecting to Michigan's Upper Peninsula, a bunch of states crammed together in the Northeast, the Dakotas abutting Minnesota. Each state had different ideas of what would work; each state had its own system for deciding when things should open and close. We were going to need public transparency and accountability for when states would reopen.

Crowdsourcing Pandemic Management

Ryan Panchadsaram, John's chief of staff, texted one day to ask if we could talk about an idea he and I had previously tossed back and forth. Ryan talked about creating a public scorecard on each state's progress: cases, hospitalizations, testing, and contact tracing. My relationship with Ryan actually predated mine with John. Ryan, who lived in San Francisco, had been a core part of the Healthcare .gov turnaround team, where everyone called him "Ryan P." A former Microsoft product manager, he'd been dogged at ferreting out undiscovered problems with Healthcare.gov, often contacting individuals who'd had problems with the site and tracing their issues all the way down to a new undiscovered problem. I began calling him the "chief curiosity officer."[1]

Ryan's idea was to build an open-source scorecard filled with everything the public needed to know about how a state was doing on public health measures. Any reasonable administration would have already made this material publicly available through the CDC. (Of course, a better administration would not have abandoned its post.) But we had "federalism" without even the basic tools the states or the public needed. I had suggested Ryan talk with the United States of Care team: Mark McClellan, who had run both CMS and the FDA and was now at Duke University, and former CDC director Tom Frieden. Together they could build a credible dashboard.

After Birx's press conference, the phone call I received from Kushner, and Trump's tweet making it clear the states were going to be left on their own, I hoped Ryan was going to tell me he had something ready. He was, in fact, calling to say that not only would he be able to launch a scorecard, but he could take Birx's criteria and use them to make a heat map and a public website that would give details of how each state was doing, what stage it was at, and what needed to happen to make progress. Ryan moves fast. By the next day—April 17, a day after the press conference—Ryan sent me a link to the first draft of the website, Covid Exit Strategy (covidexitstrategy.org).[2]

The first thing I noticed was that no state met the criteria of being ready to open, and wouldn't be ready for some time, yet many were still announcing plans to open in May.

And one other thing looked wrong immediately: every state was behind where it needed to be to open except one—the state that so far had had more than 20,000 deaths, New York. I called Ryan.

"How could New York be the state closest to being ready to reopen, Ryan? Look at the massive death toll. No one will believe that."

"It's what the data says, Andy. They are rocking on testing. They are the only ones close to meeting the White House standard."

Ryan loved data. But I didn't want him to embarrass himself.

"No one will buy this," I warned.

"No, New York is doing really well."

"Tell that to New Yorkers."

"They'll see it. It's the South I'm really worried about."

I suggested that either his data or his criteria might be wrong. But as it turned out, it was me who was wrong. Just as quickly as New York's cases had surged, they began receding, and I got a basic lesson on how the time lag between when infections begin and when the severe cases become visible could be deceiving. It's a lesson that subsequently eluded many governors.

What happened in New York? The state was actually following Italy's curve, as Birx had predicted the whole country would. Governor Cuomo had made investments in testing and contact tracing. But it was more than that. Everyone in New York City knew someone who'd had COVID-19 or been sick themselves. Many had lost friends and family. They had the sound of wailing sirens and the images of mass burials and portable morgues seared into their brains. New Yorkers had joined that fraternity of other places around the globe, such as Hong Kong, that had experienced deadly pandemics.[3] Ryan saw this happening in the data.

Ryan's map showed New Jersey and Connecticut following similar curves. But if things were going well in the Northeast, the states in the South, particularly Florida, Texas, and Arizona, were about to head in a different direction. Their Republican governors seemingly believed they had avoided the COVID-19 pandemic. None understood that it was only a matter of time until it reached them. A common refrain on the political right at the time was that the coronavirus was a blue-state and big-city problem, and people in rural America didn't need to worry.

By the end of April, instead of behaving like a unified country, in which lessons from one place would be absorbed in other places, we had southern states opening up rapidly and with few precautions. The governors wanted to see their economies bounce back, and because they hadn't experienced what New York had, they assumed they had done it better. Never mind that they hadn't met any of

Birx's suggested guidelines for reductions in cases, adequate testing, and sufficient contact tracing.

I often chatted with Chris Cuomo on his prime-time CNN show in April and May. Not only was Chris the New York governor's brother, but he was also fighting a difficult case of COVID-19 himself for much of that time. When the White House Task Force was sidelined, many of the things they were working on, like a plan to increase testing, were mothballed, and Chris wanted to know what was going to happen without federal oversight and not enough diagnostic testing needed to open the country. On his May 7 show, I warned that we were not adequately preparing to make it through the summer and fall.[4] We had chosen instant gratification over an approach that would solve the problem.

"[This] is not impossible," I said. "We need a little patience, and we need to do the real work. You can't quit in the middle. You can't announce a program to test people like we did three weeks ago and then three weeks later, when it's not done, just give up."

But giving up is what I saw everywhere. Rather than follow the guidelines Birx laid out, many states just wanted to put the whole thing behind them like it was a bad dream. Republicans I talked to, including former HHS secretary Mike Leavitt and former FDA commissioners Scott Gottlieb and Mark McClellan, told me it was fairly pointless to talk to most Republican governors about anything except economic growth. My concern was that, just as I had failed to see New York's progress, governors would fail to see the problem until it was too late. I wrote on Twitter about the optical illusion we were about to witness, and my tweets were reprinted by *Medium* on the last day of April:[5]

Welcome to 30 days of bliss. The type of bliss that often comes from ignorance. Many of the politicians in the country believe it will not be possible to keep strict social distancing rules in May. They feel pressure from a small minority to make adjustments—so people can get haircuts, gather on beaches, go to church in person, visit malls, etc. The 30 days will be blissful because people won't pay the price for May's experiment until June. But if people believe we are opening during a time when the curve is flat, they are wrong.

We are continually going to be looking at lagging data. Today we are seeing the results of early to mid-April. If you get infected today, at a minimum you'll likely experience 5 infectious days without symptoms, and 28 infectious days without symptoms for those who never show them. [Note: Subsequent studies showed that the most infectious period tapered off after approximately 10 days.] Without tests or contact tracing, you can infect many people before you know it (if you ever know it).

COVID-19 hasn't stopped being infectious just because we've socially isolated. Nothing magic happened while we were home. Pick a part of the country that hasn't done social distancing in April, prisons. The Bureau of Prisons just tested 2,000 prisoners and found 70% tested positive. In addition to being ashamed, we should be warned. The virus has gone nowhere. It is waiting us out.

On Memorial Day, we could still be looking at what could appear to be positive data that doesn't account for this lag. We might even view Memorial Day as an opportunity to celebrate together at beaches and BBQs. I know I would like that. And while most people will likely remain cautious, there's an increasing number of people who think to themselves, "If someone dies, it probably won't be me. I'm healthy and young." A new analysis today shows people dying of COVID-19 do so on average 10 years prematurely.

The Birx White House plan called for declining cases and testing and tracing, but Trump and many governors of both parties don't want to wait. They don't want to be the bad guys, don't want to deliver an uncomfortable message.

The White House Task Force remained sidelined and wouldn't publicly meet again until June 25, a full seven weeks after its last meeting.

Meanwhile, Birx was chirping about how swimmingly things were going, but Ryan's Covid Exit Strategy data showed the opposite.[6] Who was right?

States would require more than just good data to open safely. Testing, contract tracing, and isolation space for people who were infected were basic requirements when you were dealing with an infectious disease. Yet those weren't resources the states could simply create at any reasonable scale without help from the federal government.

Scott Gottlieb and I co-authored a comprehensive proposal, with support from the country's leading epidemiologists, that would create a contact tracing workforce and resources to open the economy safely. If new cases could be found and contained, the country could open and minimize the size of outbreaks. When we introduced it, the House reacted favorably, including it in the next bill they passed. Republicans in the Senate, however, looked askance at additional spending during the pandemic beyond their early bills, and they did not put forward a serious counterproposal to the House.

While Republicans were generally reluctant to spend money to fight the crisis, Democrats viewed COVID-19 the way Republicans might view a war on the American people. Democrats as conservative as Doug Jones, as progressive as Bernie Sanders, and everywhere in between called me at all hours, to talk about what could be done and how they could help.

But money wasn't the White House's concern with our contact tracing proposal. Politics was. At the end of April, I called Kushner to ask if the administration would support it. After all, it was a foundational element in the White House plan Birx had introduced.

Kushner's response was lukewarm. "It depends on how the civil liberties crowd reacts to it," he told me. I understood that to mean the Charles Koch–backed "don't tread on me" crowd on the political right that populated Trump's rallies and who were against any forceful public health measures. Trump's team wasn't going to do anything that would diminish the president's appeal among his base—they wouldn't be pushing masks, closing large gatherings, or investing in contact tracing.

Yet Trump was bothered by higher case counts—not because of

the pandemic, but because he believed the numbers reflected negatively on him. Later in the year, after boasting to a crowd about how much testing the country was doing, he would say, "Here's the bad part: when you do testing to that extent, you're gonna find more people, you're gonna find more cases. So I said to my people, slow the testing down, please!"[7] Of course, less testing meant we would have less visibility into where the virus was spreading. But that wasn't Trump's concern.

Sidelining the task force in the spring, as cases were beginning to surge in the South and West, was consistent with Trump's dismissive approach to the spread of the virus earlier in the year. In June, I wrote on Twitter, "It almost entirely goes without saying that states are on their own here. Trump has gone from 'hoax' in February to 'it's dying out' in June. It was malpractice to leave us unprepared once. It is almost a war crime to do it twice."[8] At this point, now that we understood more about how COVID-19 spread, I was sure each of these decisions would come back to haunt many in the White House as the summer wore on.

#OpenSafely . . .

As states opened up, Mark McClellan, FDA commissioner in the George W. Bush administration, and I were sure there would be trouble. We decided to shift toward helping guide people on what was safe to do and how to be careful if you lived in a state that was opening up. After all, just because your governor tells you you *can* do something doesn't mean you *should* do it.

Mark felt that helping the states figure out how to open safely might be yesterday's problem, as many states had already opened. We discussed the next problem: What would inevitably happen when cases grew, hospitals filled, and people began to die in the southern states. How would we be able to persuade southern governors that an important part of opening meant being prepared to close again?

"What would convince a governor to close their doors again?" I asked Mark.

"Well, it won't be the case count, because it will be easy to see new cases as primarily affecting a bunch of 20- and 30-year-olds, who are at lower risk of complications." The link between 30-year-olds getting infected and the spread widening to affect everyone would be too difficult to convince governors of.

"I don't even think it will be deaths," I replied. I was shaking my head, because it was hard to believe that the country was going to accept thousands of deaths because of governors who didn't understand and a president who didn't care. "Are states even paying attention to the opening criteria?"

Mark suggested that the most practical thing was to focus governors on the state of intensive care units in their states' hospitals. And indeed, from the summer through the fall, the filling up of ICUs turned out to be the only thing that would consistently capture the interest of many governors or the public. "It's a little bit risky, because if you pull the trigger too late you could be in trouble, but if you start to see case growth and the ICUs are starting to fill to a 50–60 percent level, that's when governors need to dial back on reopening."

To get a precise analysis, we turned to Caitlin Rivers, an epidemiologist at Johns Hopkins. To me, she was like the hero in the movie *Contagion*—the young, smart, adventurous epidemiologist. There was one difference: the danger she was fighting wasn't the virus itself, but ignorance about the virus. Given that governors—Republican and Democratic alike—should never have opened their states up as they did, Rivers provided the analysis we could offer governors to help them know when to pull back.

With the help of Mark McClellan, Caitlin Rivers, and many of the best epidemiologists, we put forward a consensus guide along the lines of #StayHome, with a set of rules of the road to help states and the public navigate this new terrain. We called it #OpenSafely. It was published in *USA Today* on May 20 with the headline "Health Leaders: We Stuck Together to #StayHome, Now We Can Start

Together to #OpenSafely." The piece listed activities that could be done safely as well as those that should be avoided, and it was accompanied by a set of resources for governors, mayors, and the public from United States of Care and Covid Exit Strategy.[9] Here is the opening:

Americans want our country to open up safely.

We have been at this for a number of difficult weeks since the global coronavirus pandemic began, and it has taken a toll.

It has been a time of unprecedented challenge. To our health. To our jobs. To our social connections. To our health care communities.

We have sacrificed with great unity to #StayHome in order to reduce the infection rate and save lives.

We want a sense of normalcy back—to go to work, to go to restaurants, to see sports again, to send our kids to school, to hug our families—but not at the expense of the lives of our friends, families and neighbors.

We want a good economy and public safety, but we are afraid if we open too quickly, or don't have plans to adjust if spread recurs, we will have neither.

We don't believe we need to wait until everything is completely perfect or there is zero risk before we open again. The reality is that many states are already taking the first steps toward opening, and this must happen in the safest way possible.

Americans should still #StayHome whenever possible and continue social distancing. Now we need to get on a path to #OpenSafely that gets it right.

. . . No, Just Open

When June came, we swapped our sweatpants for shorts and opened windows for welcome fresh air. Stuck inside for months in the cold Minnesota spring, I understood how badly the country just wanted it all to be over. And with reported case counts temporarily dropping, it wasn't hard to convince yourself that it was over. But it wasn't.

In fact, the virus had barely begun its invasion. By the end of May 2020, even with more than 100,000 people already dead, estimates from COVIDView, a weekly summary the CDC released, were that still well under 10 percent of the population had been infected.[10]

Our #OpenSafely guidelines reinforced the fact that there were safe and less safe ways of doing things. But they were also an attempt to hold together a consensus against the forces causing the country to come apart at the seams. In that, our efforts certainly failed. The country grew more divided as Trump remained maskless and silent about the virus, and Republican state and local officials and some in the media viewed a focus on the pandemic as left-wing hysteria designed to take down Trump.

As Mark McClellan and I had predicted, the southern states decided to learn the hard way about the virus—from their own experience. It felt like February and March all over again. We were squandering time, with a president in denial now joined by a good bit of the country. We were headed in the wrong direction, and when that happens, the problem compounds exponentially each day. Closing bars during a pandemic is like wearing a condom: it works better if you put it on before the action starts.

As we looked at states across the country, we saw that those with warmer climates were experiencing the opposite of what Trump had predicted when he said the summer heat would make the virus go away. In places where the heat forced people into air-conditioned indoor areas during the warmest months, case counts took off.[11] The aerosolization that Mike Osterholm had warned me about in March was a more significant culprit than people knew.

As temperatures and case counts rose in the South, I made a point to begin outreach to governors in northern states, where I figured we could still prepare for the moment when frigid temperatures would do in that region the same thing the sweltering summer heat had done in the South: force people inside, into poorly circulating air. Kristin Wikelius, the senior policy director at United States of Care, put together a document we sent to every state on how to prepare for the next wave. As the White House abandoned the bully pulpit, I spent my days with governors, their staffs, mayors, school superintendents, and members of Congress worried about their states. All told, I worked with 22 states, looking over plans, doing press conferences, providing input, and reviewing data. If a private company called me for help, however, I would politely decline (with the exception of the NBA, which was creating a no-profit open-source test). And I never took payment for anything. When I was offered a contract to be a pundit on CNN, I turned it down. We donated all of the profit from our podcast to relief funds for some of the hardest-hit places, including tribal reservations and farm labor camps.

Ryan put together a number of important analyses, as did modelers from other groups, such as Covid Act Now. These studies showed how delaying the implementation of mask mandates and bar closures was associated with increased cases. On May 20, we sent analyses to every governor and the mayor of every major city showing the significant benefit of early action. Too few changed their approaches, but facing a rising sea of vocal doubters, even many elected officials who didn't make changes were silently grateful for someone publicly pushing them to do the right things.

Ryan's analyses were the best amalgamations of data the country had, but he could only work with the data that was being made available. And some states were resistant to making data on infections in their state publicly available. Florida's Republican governor, Ron DeSantis, fired one of his top health data managers, Rebekah Jones, when she objected to removing crucial COVID-19 infection data from the state's website.[12] As DeSantis strutted around like a peacock in early May bragging about his state's low levels of infection, Ryan's data showed that a tsunami of cases, hospitalizations, and deaths would soon crash down on the state. Unmoved, DeSantis suppressed the release of the data and refused to take action until June 26, by which time the state was seeing more than 5,000 new cases per day, almost five times the number it had seen in May. When he finally deputized the secretary of the state's Department of Business and Professional Regulation to tweet that Florida bars would be closing, it was already too late. By summer's end, Florida would have more than 15,700 deaths. And yet DeSantis would again reopen the bars precipitously in September.[13]

DeSantis never called me, but members of Florida's congressional delegation did, a number of times. My suggestion to them was to galvanize the hospitality industry around sacrificing now if they wanted to open tourism for the holiday tourist season. Doing so would mean taking matters into their own hands by closing bars, urging mask wearing, and issuing the most stringent rules on gatherings. They organized a call for me to speak to hotel and tourism representatives on August 11. Not surprisingly, they wanted to stay open now *and* have full hotels in December.

I delivered the tough news. "Nobody ever said in a pandemic you could have everything. You have to pick the least bad option: bars in the summer or hope for a tourist season in December. You choose," I told them.

Without more congressional support, few businesses were in a financial position to make difficult sacrifices. Mitch McConnell was sitting on a proposal from the House that included loans to hard-hit businesses, money for small businesses and nonprofits (including targeted assistance to restaurants and live-performance venues), one year's worth of assistance to state governments, and expanded unemployment benefits. He was refusing to act on it, leaving places like Florida with only bad options.[14] I felt for the business owners in Florida. Their suffering was real, and they weren't being offered great choices. But things didn't bode well for the holidays.

In the chaos, getting someone to act early enough was difficult. In Arizona, Republican governor Doug Ducey lifted the stay-at-home order on May 15, 2020. By May 26, cases started to increase.[15] On June 8, my friend Peter Fine, the CEO of Banner Health, the largest hospital system in the state, rang the alarm about the increasing number of people needing ICU treatment, but the governor ignored him. On June 11, I received a call from Ruben Gallego, the Democratic congressman for Arizona's 7th District, which includes Phoenix and Scottsdale. He wanted help staving off the surge. On June 15, Gallego and I held a press conference in which we tried to persuade the governor to temporarily close bars and ask people to wear masks.[16] For the next 10 days, cases continued to grow and hospitals were in crisis. On June 25, after a month of doing nothing, Governor Ducey called a press conference in which he said, "The rate of the spread of this virus is unacceptable," and encouraged people to wear masks, but refused to mandate it, or to close bars and restaurants. Two days earlier, he had attended an indoor campaign rally for Trump in Phoenix—where, to his credit, he was one of the very few people wearing a mask.[17]

Finally, on June 29, Ducey closed bars, restaurants, and movie theaters and limited public gatherings. On June 30, Arizona reached its highest number of reported cases in a single day, nearly 4,800, and then the case count began to drop. By the end of the summer, 5,700 people had died in the state.[18] Ducey waited until the speedboat was nearly out of sight to start swimming.

All across the country, a national failure to prepare had become a failure to adapt. This would end up being the story of June and July, as governors were left on their own to decide how to respond to things. Each decision—when to close bars, when to require masks, when to issue stay-at-home orders—had a direct impact on the death toll. Not closing the bars for another weekend meant more lives would be lost. Waiting a week on a mask order meant more lives lost.

Across the board, governors sensed how weary the people in their states were of the virus. Politicians all want to be liked. So putting place restrictions no one liked was a litmus test for political courage. After just a couple of phone conversations and a look at the data, Jacob Frey, the mayor of Minneapolis, decided to close indoor bars during the middle of summer. But other public officials had a variety of rationalizations for not acting. Among them were a few, such as South Dakota governor Kristi Noem, who believed in taking a "freedom-first" strategy instead of asking people to wear masks.[19] The result? South Dakota became the world's hot spot. There were days in the fall when more than half of the people tested in South Dakota were positive for COVID-19.[20]

The Scientist Breaks Free

In person, Deborah Birx was tough, smart, and confident in a way she couldn't demonstrate in a briefing with a president who wouldn't be shown up. When she lost all ability to persuade him, she began touring the country instead, and tried to persuade states to take more extreme measures.[21] She wanted all bars closed, mask mandates, and an end to large gatherings. She traveled with reams and reams of data and visited state capitals, colleges, and cities, looking at compliance with these directives and comparing them to the data she saw. All smiles on TV, she could get angry making her point. (The Trump administration kept these reports confidential even though they contained the best clues for the public on where the virus was spreading. During the first week of the Biden administration, we made these reports public.)

The problem, of course, was that she was advocating for the opposite of what her boss was insisting on. Still, Birx grew more and more concerned over the summer and fall of 2020, pointing to Memorial Day and Independence Day, with all of their gatherings, as times when the virus had spread to new places and hot spots sprang up. As she traveled, she pushed the responsibility onto governors, colleges, local health departments, vacationers, people who flouted masking rules—anywhere but the president.

Through the White House, Birx had access to highly detailed information about case growth, risks, and threats. The problem was that she was not permitted to make the information public in a visible way. So she used her travels to dribble it out the best she could. Still, she was being undermined by the FDA and CDC, whose messaging was being directed by the White House (I will detail that in Chapter 10).

In August, I confronted her on the challenge of being contradicted by the president. The CDC, now directed by Trump political appointees, had put out guidelines telling people who were asymptomatic that they didn't need to get tested—one of the many things that flew in the face of her guidance. "The concern now for the FDA and CDC [putting out false information] is real," I said to her. "How [do] you guide people when that messaging is so contrary to what a lot of the local public health officials and clinicians are telling them?"

She responded, "This is why this week we'll have our tenth governors' report. It's very specific. . . . We've decided to work directly with every single state and mayor, to really get the information out. We've been calling for surveillance testing at universities, in the governors' report, for the last two months [in contrast to the CDC]."

As much as Birx said "we," she was going rogue. And she would pay the price: by August 10, she had effectively been replaced as the scientific advisor to the president by Scott Atlas, a man with no qualifications other than an opinion Trump agreed with, which was that the entire pandemic was just wildly overblown.[22] But at least Birx was out there focusing on saving the next life.

Unfortunately, state success rates were highly variable. On any given day, Ryan's website showed that in at least half of the states the outlook was declining—a condition he marked with the color red. Some days 49 out of 50 states bore this mark of shame. (He even had to add another color, called "bruised red," to his national map as things worsened.) Birx's efforts were simply no substitute for a comprehensive national approach.

To compound the problems of the summer, after a poor start, the country still didn't have enough diagnostic testing. The flood of new cases was making rapid testing essential given the fact that people can become contagious 48 to 72 hours before experiencing symptoms. I received a disturbing call from the secretary of health in North Carolina, Mandy Cohen, my former chief of staff at CMS, to let me know they were experiencing a backlog of seven days to get test results. Because of this, on any day the new positive cases being publicly reported weren't a true reflection of actual infections at that time.

Meanwhile, there was nobody watching the store. No active task force meant no focus. I tweeted, "We are back to where we were in March when we didn't have enough tests." I tried to lay out our choices in very simple terms.[23]

> If cases keep growing, it is not possible to scale testing exponentially. So we as a society have a few choices to make.
> - Going to bars or working to open schools
> - Pushing employees back to work or WFH
> - Fighting over masks vs wearing one
> - Continuing to go state by state or pushing the fed government to take more responsibility

In early July, cases were growing exponentially again, this time not by 30,000 cases a day but by 70,000.[24] We learned how badly Birx had miscalculated in April in comparing the United States to Italy: from mid-May through the summer, the United States had four times the death rate of Italy.[25]

On July 11, Adam Boehler told his staff at the U.S. International Development Finance Corporation that he would be headed back to the White House.

"I've just been dealing with the Taliban," he said to me later. "They're an easier enemy than COVID."

CHAPTER 8

THE ROOM SERVICE PANDEMIC

SCENE: THE UNEXAMINED CORNERS OF OUR COUNTRY

> It really boils down to this: that all life is interrelated. We are all caught in an inescapable network of mutuality, tied into a single garment of destiny. Whatever affects one directly, affects all indirectly. We are made to live together because of the interrelated structure of reality.
>
> —Martin Luther King Jr., Christmas Eve 1967[1]

Each morning before the sun was fully up, Ahmed Aden arrived at the warehouse where he worked, got on the elevator, pressed the button, and rode down to his underground workstation, where he scanned packages for delivery.

It was April 2020, and the Amazon warehouse in Minnesota where Ahmed worked was busier than it had been since Christmas. He worked long days packing up orders for people who had the luxury of working from their homes. Each night he returned to his two-bedroom apartment, where his wife, Safia, prepared dinner for him and their seven kids. Ahmed had been the last of the family to arrive in America from a refugee camp in Addis Ababa, and he was reluctant to speak English with his more fluent wife and children.

Almost all the employees at the Amazon warehouse were Somali immigrants like him. He had never received a package from Amazon himself, but he liked to imagine people opening the packages he loaded into the trucks, filled with video games, books, electric toothbrushes, new TVs, and Bluetooth speakers. He took pride in being one of the people keeping the country moving. As an essential worker, he considered his job important. His pay did not cover all of the family's modest expenses, but one of his daughters, Rahma, worked at a local pharmacy and was able to contribute.

By March 30, several of Ahmed's co-workers had called in sick, including Cumar, the older man with the cough who worked at the station next to his. On April 6, about a week after Cumar stopped coming to work, Ahmed learned that he was in the hospital. That same day Ahmed began experiencing symptoms while on the job. By the time he left the warehouse in the afternoon, he was shaking, sweating through his shirt, and coughing. When he got home, Safia took one look at him and knew the virus she'd been following on the news was now in his body.

Quarantining in their crowded apartment was a challenge. Safia put him in their bedroom, and she and the five children who still lived at home crammed into the other bedroom. Their youngest son, Hassan, age 15, had cerebral palsy and required her constant care. The stores in their neighborhood were sold out of household cleaning supplies, so Safia gathered all the soap in the house, diluted it with water, and scrubbed every wall and surface as soon as her children were asleep. A year into treatment for breast cancer, which had weakened her immune system, Safia knew catching the virus would be especially dangerous for her.

After his two paid weeks of sick leave, Ahmed had to take another month off from work, unpaid, because he was too sick to leave his bed. Safia worried they would soon run out of money. To make matters worse, Rahma didn't want to go back to work at the pharmacy and risk spreading the virus to customers. She believed it was proper for her to isolate, so she told her manager that she needed to stay home. He told her she would not be paid unless she could show that she'd tested positive for COVID-19. But no tests were available. She chose to isolate in their small apartment anyway, even though she too lost her paycheck.

After three weeks, two of Ahmed's daughters were also sick. Ahmed went with them to the county hospital for tests, and all were positive. Because the other members of his family were not presenting symptoms, they were not able to get tests. Miraculously, Hassan and Safia remained healthy. It would be another five weeks before Ahmed would be well enough to leave the bedroom. The day after that, desperate for money to support his family, he returned to the warehouse.

▪▪▪

"I don't know anyone who has died of COVID-19."

It wasn't the only time I had heard this, and I detected a mild accusation beneath the comment. If I don't know anyone, how could it be true? I was on a Zoom call at the request of a friend, talking with a group of his clients about the state of the pandemic.

Millions of Americans have never been to Albania, but few doubt the country exists. Denying the threat from the coronavirus demonstrated more than just a lack of imagination. This was a lack of a certain kind of imagination.

"That's because you don't know the people who grow your food. Or deliver it to the stores. Or stock the shelves. Or deliver it to your house," I replied. "These people work for you; you just don't know their names." I didn't bother to mention county jails, homeless shelters, immigrant detention centers, or public housing.

Our Moral Test

Every weekday for two and a half years, I walked to work by cutting across the Washington Mall in front of the U.S. Capitol to the Hubert H. Humphrey Building, a Brutalist monster made of cinder block and brick featuring narrow windows that, amazingly, offered no view of the U.S. Capitol across the street. After passing through security, HHS workers and visitors find themselves in an overly large lobby, a cavernous box with 35-foot ceilings in what can only be a government building, one that could just as easily be in Beijing or Moscow. High on one of the walls is a quotation from Hubert Humphrey, the Minnesotan who served as vice president to Lyndon Johnson.[2] It reads:

> The moral test of government is how that government treats those who are in the dawn of life, the children; those who are in the twilight of life, the elderly; and those who are in the shadows of life, the sick, the needy and the handicapped.

Each morning I passed underneath that quote on the way to my office on the third floor. Humphrey's words were true in the 1960s, when Medicare and Medicaid were passed into law and began to transform the lives of millions of older and low-income Americans; they remained true when the Children's Health Insurance Program became law in 1997 and the Affordable Care Act became law in 2010.[3] And during the global pandemic of 2020 and beyond, there may not be a more apt and important sentiment.

But beginning in 2017, a very different vision prevailed at HHS. Alex Azar and his team oversaw a series of policies that directly challenged Humphrey's vision. They allowed children crossing into the United States from Mexico to be separated from their parents and kept in cages at detention centers. They overturned a rule protecting LGBTQ Americans from discrimination when they seek health care. They discouraged immigrants from using their legally granted benefits. Under orders from the White House, they prohibited diversity and inclusion training for staffers. And they illegally attempted to deny Medicaid coverage to some low-income Americans, instructing them to find better work or else lose access to their coverage. All these actions were part of a philosophy of governing that was wed to both an Ayn Rand–style capitalist doctrine and a conservative religious doctrine and was outwardly hostile to the federal government's prominent role in health care.[4]

In Trump's HHS, the words *health* and *human services* themselves lost their meaning, except in an Orwellian sense. Under Trump and Azar, the Office of Civil Rights, a congressionally mandated part of HHS since 1966, reversed its mission of protecting people who were discriminated against, and was converted into an office to protect people who believed their Christian faith forbade them from caring for anyone they had a moral objection to. All this took place underneath the watchful words of Humphrey.[5]

In 2020, as the human tragedy of the pandemic was unfolding, the death toll was being felt the most strongly in precisely the places where Humphrey had placed our moral test. Veterans' homes, jails, nursing homes, detention centers, farm labor camps, homeless shelters, and cramped public housing were where the virus did its worst damage. Through mid-November, the death rate in the Black community was 110 per 100,000 people, more than twice the rate for Whites. One out of every 1,429 Black Americans had been killed by COVID-19 before the fall of 2020 even began.[6]

People like Ahmed—people who needed to work every day so that their families could eat, many of whom lacked health insurance or ready access to a doctor or medicine—faced the risks of the pandemic every day. Others, who lived in the homes where Ahmed's packages went, faced much lower risks, and soon became eager to get on with their lives.

Whom Are We Asking to Die?

In the first six months of the pandemic, I often heard the same questions over and over: *Why* are so many Americans being allowed to die? *What* are we doing wrong? *How* could we have gotten it so wrong? One aspect of the U.S. response can be explained by looking at a different question: *Who* is being hurt the most?

In Texas, a state that doesn't believe much in central government, the lieutenant governor's role is unlike that in any other state. In many ways, the Texas lieutenant governor is more powerful than the governor. He is president of the State Senate and also leads the Legislative Budget Board, where he controls the budgeting process. The lieutenant governor regularly participates in the legislative process and has the power to create committees and appoint committee chairs and members. And the lieutenant governor is elected independently of the governor, so he is in no way politically obliged to follow the governor's lead—either in matters of policy or in how he conducts himself.

Dan Patrick, a former AM radio host, became Texas's 42nd lieutenant governor in January 2015. Early in his career he changed his name from Dannie Scott Goeb and became a sports broadcaster. Even though he was from Baltimore, Maryland, he took to wearing a large cowboy hat. He developed a reputation for arrogance. After an early career covering sports, he tried to parlay his notoriety into a chain of sports bars, which went bankrupt, leaving his creditors holding the bag for several hundred thousand dollars in debt. He then returned to radio as a conservative commentator, where he found more success. His most notable achievement is having helped launch Rush Limbaugh's career.[7]

Patrick made his bones igniting the culture wars. Guns, God, and hate for immigrants were Patrick's can't-miss issues, but opposing rights for LGBTQ Americans was another one of his favorites. In 2016, he received national attention for this pseudo-biblical tweet following the mass shooting at Pulse, a gay nightclub in Orlando, Florida: "Do not be deceived. God cannot be mocked. A man reaps what he sows."[8] He once used a gay slur to describe fellow Texas politician Beto O'Rourke.[9]

Patrick was a frequent guest on Fox News programs because of his penchant for controversy. He stoked the political right and baited liberals, doubling his chances for a viral clip. During the pandemic, as the country adapted to social distancing restrictions, Patrick opined to Tucker Carlson that "there are more important things than living. And that's saving the country for my children and my grandchildren. . . . We got to take some risks and get back in the game, and get this country back up and running."[10] The clip received more than 400,000 views.

Patrick spoke for a lot of people that day, particularly those who felt their personal risk of dying from coronavirus was low but that the damage to the economy could actually hurt them. For some people living in communities behind guarded gates—from Houston, Texas, to the Villages in Florida, and including governors' mansions throughout much of the South—Patrick had said out loud and bluntly what many of them were feeling.

Beto O'Rourke, the El Paso–born and raised politician Patrick had derided, was his polar opposite. A skateboard-riding former punk rock guitarist and popular past congressman, O'Rourke was tall and engaging, with a knack for appealing to people's inner decency. These traits and his millennial star power made him a successful campaigner and drove people like Patrick crazy.

During the pandemic, O'Rourke and I talked and texted regularly, particularly as deaths in border communities spiked. In May he framed for me one of the central questions of the pandemic: "Our lieutenant governor on Fox said that there are some things that are more important than living. And that then begs the question, who then is he asking to do the dying?[11]

"In a state like Texas," O'Rourke went on, "where the minimum wage is $7.25 an hour, those we are sending into harm's way when these retail shops reopen are, by and large, the working poor. There's a bartender who lives down the block from me. And the week that the state was set to reopen, we happened to be walking our dog by his house. And he said, 'Hey, Beto, I just got a call to go back to work this week. And I'm really struggling because I need the income. I won't be able to collect unemployment if I refuse the offer from my boss, but my wife really doesn't want me to go back. We have a young child, we have older parents, and I'm really struggling with the decision.' I think he ended up not going into work and is, I guess, going to try to find some way to meet the payment on his mortgage note and put food on the table in his house."

Over the summer, the border communities in Texas, particularly along the Rio Grande Valley, faced a crisis. In rural communities, hospitals were small and not well equipped for patients in need of intensive care. By Independence Day, Starr County's only hospital was at capacity. Neighboring Cameron County's hospitals were also turning patients away. Ambulances were parked in front of hospitals and used as beds; even the crematoriums had long waiting lists. Patients were dying, and some of the small number of providers were falling ill. But outside the spotlight of a city like Houston or Dallas, these developments got very little attention. In normal circumstances, a crisis of this magnitude alone would be worthy of national news attention, support from FEMA, and doctors and nurses flying in on voluntary missions from all over the country. But not now. As I talked to people in local hospitals, to O'Rourke, and to Peter Hotez, a Texas-based infectious disease specialist, it was clear that Texas's governor, Greg Abbott, wasn't doing much of anything about it.

Early in the morning on July 25, I called and left a message for the White House Task Force asking for help. When they called me back, I learned that they were not even aware of the situation in Texas. Even at this point in the summer, with more than 1,000 deaths a day across the country and cases at an all-time high, I had the sense that the White House felt people were exaggerating how bad things were—and that there was an alternative way of looking at the situation that wasn't as troubling.

The person I spoke to at the White House asked me, "Are these people coming across the border?"

"That's what people do in border towns," I replied. "That's how the economy works there."

It felt like they wanted to know if the people falling ill were "real Americans" before they would consider pursuing my suggestion to airlift patients to bigger cities. The best I could do was persuade them to look at the data and call the governor's office. They did, and were told the situation in the Rio Grande Valley was being grossly exaggerated.

I contacted one of Governor Abbott's advisors and heard something similar. People in Abbott's administration believed local Democratic officials were out to make the governor look bad. "Remember, these local judges [who made municipal decisions in Texas] have vendettas against Abbott, so I wouldn't take their word at face value," the advisor told me.

By October, 3,000 people in the valley were dead. By November, El Paso couldn't procure any more portable freezers for the bodies. Worse, that death toll was hardly noticed outside the immediate area. Communities like those along the border in Texas were especially easy to ignore. And such invisible communities—home to day laborers, immigrants, homeless populations, foster children—were everywhere, but the media seldom took us there. I spent a number of days and nights talking to governors, sharing Ryan P.'s data with them, hoping to shed light and bring resources wherever possible. Most of the time, I was not successful. But as hopeless as the effort may have been, I couldn't stop.

One lesson on how the virus worked and who was at risk was in the damage it could do in places where there was no escape from close quarters. In Cook County Jail in Chicago, the first two cases were diagnosed on March 23, 2020. By April 8, 238 of the 4,500 inmates had tested positive, as had 115 guards and other staff—many of whom returned home to infect their family members when their shifts ended. The vast majority of the inmates had still not been tested, and yet the jail was the largest known source of infection in the country at that time.[12] In the United States in 2020, 2.3 million people are behind bars, not counting those in immigration detention centers.[13] In California's San Quentin prison, 2,000 cases had been reported among approximately 3,300 inmates by July 23, and 15 of them had died.[14]

And it's not just prisons where the toll from the coronavirus is being largely ignored:

- Homeless shelters found that 18–30 percent or more of their residents are testing positive for COVID-19.[15]
- In South Dakota, where the governor refused to take any safety measures to protect the public, there were 644 cases at one meatpacking plant.[16]

- On May 18, the Navajo Nation surpassed New York State for the highest infection rate; by mid-October 2020, there were 10,696 reported cases and 565 deaths.[17] There are several reasons for the rampant spread of the disease in the Navajo Nation.[18] Phone service is limited and it can take hours to drive to some homes, making contact tracing difficult. Not everyone has clean running water, so it can be hard to follow the handwashing protocol. Add to this the prevalence among the Navajo population of chronic health conditions such as obesity, asthma, and diabetes, combine that with insufficient federal funding, and you have a recipe for a public health crisis.

But Dan Patrick wasn't simply condemning some people to die. He was condemning others to isolation: younger people who were sick or who had disabilities, people with compromised immune systems who still wanted to live. Poignant examples were everywhere if you looked. One of our close family friends with whom we spent many Jewish holidays had a son who had grown up and attended school with our older son, Caleb. He had been born with a heart condition and had been living immunocompromised for years. In December 2019, he came down with a lingering pneumonia. Up until that point, despite his health, he had been able to have a relatively normal existence, taking only minor precautions. But when the pandemic hit, that changed, and the entire family was forced to completely isolate to keep him safe from the virus. His mother recalled something he had told her, words that could have been spoken by so many with chronic conditions who have been sentenced to what feels like indefinite isolation. "I'm 24 years old and I'm not doing anything. I'm not in school, not working," he'd told her. "Am I going to be here until I'm 40?"[19] Sadly, even that was not to be. On April 22, 2020, at age 24, he died in his sleep of complications from his illness.

The old, the poor, and the sick were being relegated to second-class citizenship. Our real values are not the ones that disappear in hard times; they're the ones that show up in hard times. All it took was one little pandemic, and we started writing people off.

The Guarded-Gate Response

To the extent that the United States had a lockdown, I think of it as something like a "room service lockdown." On one side of the hotel room door, the pandemic didn't look so bad. As I sat in our suburban house outside of Minneapolis with enough savings to get through the pandemic, my privilege made my experience under the state's stay-at-home order very different from Ahmed's. Amazon packages, meal delivery, Netflix, Zoom meetings, and grocery delivery were easy to get for people like me. If you were privileged enough and had the income and the ability to work from home, it could be easy to be dismissive of the dangers.

And when people like me got careless, it was very often others who paid the price.

On August 7 in Millinocket, Maine, there was a wedding attended by 62 guests. After the wedding it was revealed that 10 of those guests had been infected with COVID-19. A month later at least 170 people had contracted the disease from one of those wedding guests, and 8 of them were dead. None of the deceased had attended the wedding themselves. The coronavirus had been passed on to each of them by attendees who, likely without knowing it, spread the virus to their friends, their neighbors, and people who worked near them.[20]

As Americans experienced their first pandemic in living memory, the nature of the U.S. response to COVID-19 allowed some people the luxury of believing they could ignore public health warnings. Trump's downplaying of the risks was music to their ears, as it affirmed their own reality. Many more people were likely to know someone who had lost their job as a result of the pandemic than someone who had lost their life. If you didn't know Ahmed, it was harder to have empathy for him.

If the virus didn't deeply impact your community, that reshaped your view of everything. Steps to contain outbreaks, such as contact tracing, felt like a blame game to many Americans, who resented what seemed like a challenge to their basic liberties.[21] Some families resisted getting their children tested for COVID-19 or participating in contact tracing, because parents did not want their family to be the one that caused a school to be closed.

At the same time, many well-off folks were getting tests for their own safety while not cooperating with tracing efforts. Private labs like Valley Medical Laboratory, with locations near my home in Minnesota, were offering COVID-19 tests, with results within 24 hours, for $120. Lana had a Facebook friend who took her daughter to Valley Medical and noticed that after the child tested positive she wasn't asked for contacts they could trace.[22] She asked Lana if this seemed strange. Indeed, it was. Her friend contacted the state Department of Health, and it turned out that Valley Medical was also delaying reporting test results to the state, as required by law. In essence, the clinic was doing nothing to slow the spread of the virus. While its representatives deny that was their intention, the clinic catered to the desires of its high-end customers.

The problem is not limited to Minnesota. In Massachusetts, contact tracers reported that more than half of the people they had attempted to reach by phone just didn't answer, perhaps in part because people are reluctant to answer calls from unrecognized numbers.[23] And often when the contact tracers did succeed in getting hold of someone, the person would refuse to cooperate. For example, college students and high school students who might have contracted the virus at a party they shouldn't have been at were reluctant to get their friends in trouble by saying who else was at the party with them.

Meanwhile, though, in areas with high community spread, deaths always come—though generally not to those who have felt least at risk.

Essential Workers

What was hard to see was just how wide the social gaps had become—and what our social divisions meant for the spread of the virus. While those getting the room service may have complained the loudest, those on the other side of the room service divide, like Ahmed, were the ones at higher risk. Estimates suggested that even when many people thought that almost everyone was following a strict stay-at-home order, 45 percent of Americans were required to report to work each day, many of them interacting with and serving the public: food growers, distributors, delivery personnel, retail workers, mail carriers, flight attendants, sanitation workers, plumbers, and health care workers.[24]

On July 8, I testified via Zoom at a hearing of the Minnesota House Select Committee on Pandemic Response and Rebuilding.[25] One legislator at the hearing asked whether I would support an indoor mask mandate for public places. I replied: "I would, because we have a mandate that people have to work and be around us. If someone is forced to see my face, the least I could do is put a mask on."

The more people who are required to interact with the public, the more there is an obligation to protect those workers by wearing masks.

Ahmed and his colleagues were the not-so-secret secret of the pandemic. Not only did they disproportionately pay with their health, but they were also hurt worse financially. Employment rates were down 19.7 percent for the lowest-income workers between January and September 2020, compared to a drop of 5.7 percent for middle-income workers and only 0.8 percent for high-income earners.[26]

After the Minnesota House's hearing, I laid out a brief 10-point plan for addressing the needs of essential workers, from retrofitting workplaces and transportation for safety to committing to free testing, PPE, and paid medical leave. And I wrote this on Twitter:[27]

If someone tells you that you're "essential," you're going to want to run the other way. Because "essential" now means underpaid, unappreciated, sacrificial, and there to serve everyone else.

In the future, definitions in the dictionary are going to need to include what "essential worker" came to mean during the COVID-19 crisis. You were essential, but your health, your income, your life, your safety net, and your wellbeing, it turns out, are "not as essential."

Keeping America's steaks and Big Macs was essential to Trump as he called meat packing plants essential before they could retrofit so as to not become blazing hot spots. You show who's essential by who you protect and who you don't.

Being asked to go to work to keep America moving is nothing new to people who get up early in the morning to pick crops, drive trucks, move boxes, stock shelves, ring the register and bring things to our doors.

Other countries like Italy drew much harder lines and asked for much more sacrifice from the "non-essential" than we did. Shopping only on certain days of the week. Better isolation. More short-term pain for all, for quicker long-term gain, instead of luxury for some on the shoulders of others.

A crisis shows our truest colors. The U.S. put the needs of the well-off first, asking for relatively minor sacrifice (other than learning Zoom angles and teaching math to our kids, which is actually no small thing). But "essential" workers have had it different.

Essential workers sleep on couches to reduce family spread, beg for masks, take public transport and, of course, interact with "non-essential" people who refuse to wear masks or socially distance. This just scratches the surface of the indignities of being "essential."

Black communities not only have been getting disproportionately sicker from COVID-19 but are disproportionately asked to work to support the rest of the country. Wonder if there's any correlation . . .

There's been no hazard pay, job guarantee, minimum wage (let alone Universal Basic Income), guaranteed paid sick leave. And now we are allowing people to get evicted from their apartments.

People who can't make rent in this difficult time—including many who we think of as "essential"—will be evicted along with their families. Yes, Trump campaign supporters will repeat that this is "a wonderful economy." An economy built on Amazon and GrubHub orders while food lines for the essential workers there are at record levels.

If Trump and McConnell want to run in 2020 on the economy, they should start by making it a priority to keep people safe, put money in their pockets and allow them to avoid medical debt, homelessness and hunger. That'd be a good start for someone you consider essential.

And essential workers should be reason enough for us to mask up. If it's a hardship for you to wear a mask, please don't force people who have no choice to come face-to-face with you.

Single moms with a sick kid. People who can't visit an elderly parent. Laborers with a family in a one-bedroom apartment. I hear from all of them. These are the people we don't see very well when we make policies and talk about the "essential worker." Our proud tradition of stepping up for people in need in this country in times of floods or hurricanes will instead become our own 21st-century Dickens story. If we don't do something, this is how the history of COVID-19 will be told.

Racism

When Blythe Adamson agreed to stay on at the White House, there was one project that was important to her. Surrounded by young, confident, wealthy men with thin ties and parted hair who argued for opening the country up, and by economists so eager for GDP growth, Blythe wanted to understand why so many poor people were dying, people who lived in circumstances not much different from her own not too long ago. And, in particular, she wanted to answer the question of why so many Black and Latinx people were dying. Was it their underlying health conditions, their lack of access to care, or something else?

On the morning of June 15, I had a call with Gretchen Whitmer.

The Michigan governor shared data showing that 35 percent of the COVID-19 cases in her state were among African Americans, who represented only 15 percent of the state's population. That same day, I had a call with the mayor's team in Baton Rouge, Louisiana, who were deeply concerned that the burden of COVID-19 was disproportionately falling on the same people who were facing job losses, potential homelessness, and food lines.

Cleavon Gilman, an emergency room doctor in New York and later in Arizona, told me, "The ICUs in the beginning were full of people of all races and colors. Now it's entirely Black and Brown people coming in: essential workers and their families."

As of October 2020, one-third of all Americans over the age of 65 who have been hospitalized with the virus are Black, a rate almost four times higher than the rate for White people of the same age group.[28]

There were other challenges to controlling the spread in minority communities, as Ned Lamont, the governor of Connecticut, related to me when he called in late July. "I've been hearing what you've been saying about Arizona and wondering if you're seeing any of the same trends in Connecticut?" he asked.

Fortunately, I wasn't. I checked Ryan P.'s chart of leading indicators. On May 1, Connecticut had had 30 cases for every 100,000 residents. Now, in July, that was down to 4. Even more important, his chart showed that at this point Connecticut was all green on the indicators set up by Dr. Birx and the CDC (the indicators that nobody was using, of course).

"We have another problem," Lamont said. "The Hispanic community doesn't seem to be doing contact tracing. This is one of our potential holes."

Both sides of the room service transaction were concerned about contact tracing, though for different reasons. People of color were proving highly reluctant to help contact tracers, and this was especially so for the Latinx community, as many of them feared they would be reported to U.S. Customs and Immigration Enforcement. This was the cost of the erosion of trust between the government and the community. Since anyone can spread or get the virus, it was a potent example of why our inhumane treatment of immigrants was harmful.

Even immigrants with documentation proving that they were in the country legally were being actively discouraged from using the Medicaid system or SNAP vouchers (food stamps) under a rule that came from people working in that HHS building with Hubert Humphrey's quote on the wall. It was called the "public charge rule," and it used a particularly strong point of leverage: any use of public benefits by immigrants would make their application for a green card more difficult.[29] Now, with the Latinx community dying from COVID-19 at a rapidly increasing rate, the Trump administration was discouraging them from seeking medical care and also from cooperating with authorities seeking to find out who in their community might be infected. It doesn't require genius to see how none of this was helping slow down the virus.

Furthermore, 24 percent of Latinx workers were in occupations classified as essential.[30] They held jobs including farm work, truck driving, lawn service, and food distribution. Those who worked in meatpacking were in the worst possible setting for safety: in close quarters, with loud shouting and poor ventilation. As a result, Latinx people were three times as likely to die from COVID-19 as Whites. And Black people were 3.5 times as likely to succumb to the disease. According to the Brookings Institution, Black people are dying at the same rate as White people more than 10 years older.[31]

Some occupations were particularly susceptible to COVID-19, and the country was particularly indifferent to them. There are an estimated 2.5 million agricultural workers in the country living in farm labor camps and moving from place to place as they follow the harvest.[32] They often work in the hot sun with little protection from exposure. Depending on the crop, workers may crawl along on their knees to harvest strawberries or climb 75 feet up in the air to harvest dates. About half the workers are undocumented, a result of the lack of citizen labor to meet the needs of U.S. consumers. This has the added benefit to large agribusiness of making sub-human working conditions more acceptable. As a rule, the farm owners are solidly Trump supporters, and farming is one area where the government is less than scrupulous about documentation.

For farmworkers, unemployment insurance, stimulus checks, and safety regulations are uncommon. Workers are often transported in crowded pickup trucks and trailers. The work typically requires daily movement from farm to farm and seasonal migration from community to community. The Trump administration refused to dedicate testing resources to this group of workers or impose safety regulations on their employers—even after the CDC made explicit recommendations to do so.

As of mid-October, six of the seven counties with the greatest number of COVID-19 cases per capita were in the Central Valley of California, the largest producer of fruits and vegetables in the country. Two of the other largest farm labor counties in the United States—Imperial County in California and Yuma in Arizona, both border towns—also had high infection rates.[33]

I asked the California state secretary of health and human services, Mark Ghaly, if all the cases in farm labor camps were due to field conditions, transportation, or housing. His answer? "Yes."

Unequal outcomes by race are nothing new in health care. As I mentioned in Chapter 2, health outcomes for Black people are worse across the board during non-pandemic times. Black women are 22 percent more likely to die from heart disease than White women, and 71 percent more likely to die from cervical cancer. Blacks are diagnosed with diabetes at a 71 percent higher rate than Whites. And minorities receive lower-quality care for their diabetes, resulting in more complications such as chronic kidney disease and amputations. The list of conditions from which Blacks suffer more extends to mental health, cancer, and heart disease.[34]

What plagues the U.S. health care system is not universally poor outcomes but poor outcomes for the bottom rungs of society—low-income populations and racial minorities. As with much inequality, the factors that result in this outcome feed on one another to make the problem worse.[35] Black Americans are less likely to be able to find a physician who will treat them. The physicians they do find are less likely to give them a needed prescription for pain relief, as they are more likely to be seen as "drug seekers."[36] They are also less likely to be able to afford the prescriptions they are given. They are more likely to have unaddressed trauma, often multi-generational and childhood trauma. Healthy and nutritious foods are less likely to be available in predominantly Black neighborhoods, while candy bars and alcohol and low-cost fast food are more likely to be in abundance. Consistently, studies have shown that these factors are related to race independent of income. All of this puts Black communities at higher risk of developing more severe COVID-19. So do more densely packed neighborhoods with less green space, more poorly ventilated living arrangements, and more frequent use of public transportation.

Blythe saw it in the data. During the periods of stay-at-home orders, more people of color were going to work, riding the train, and working in places with more and longer exposure to the virus.

Yes, this is known as structural racism. There's an old saying, "When America catches a cold, Black people get the flu." Well, in 2020, when America catches coronavirus, Black and Latinx people die.[37]

Seniors and People with Disabilities

In December 2017, with great fanfare, Donald Trump announced he would not be enforcing the penalties previously established for nursing homes that violated the landmark safety regulations released by the Obama administration. That set of regulations, which I proudly signed in 2016, hadn't been updated for more than a decade and weighed in at a hefty 11,000 pages, which allowed Trump to point to them as a classic example of government overreach. He saw the elimination of these safety regulations as an example of his flair for business-friendly deregulation.[38] At the time, I protested loudly, but few people noticed the issue.

There are an estimated 15,600 nursing homes in the United States, which care for 1.7 million American seniors and people with disabilities.[39] When COVID-19 hit, it hit seniors the hardest—in nursing homes, in assisted living centers, and in veterans' homes.

What I heard from people who worked in nursing homes wasn't pretty. Many had no protective gear. Staff often worked in multiple nursing homes in the same day or the same week, introducing the coronavirus into new nursing homes along the way. There were no tests available for them or for patients. Management was overwhelmed and unprepared, with neither the ventilation nor the infection control systems needed to keep residents safe. (My college friend Rob and his brother, Dave, whose father died in a New Jersey nursing home where many others died, reported that there had been no separation between their father and other residents.) As infections began ripping through nursing home after nursing home, many homes became short-staffed, as physicians and attendants were barred from entering. In some states, such as New York, this was exacerbated by policies that moved patients out of hospitals into nursing homes. (This and subsequent steps by Governor Cuomo to obfuscate his actions turned into a scandal when they were discovered in 2021.) But when the COVID-19 pandemic began, hospitals refused to take sick patients from the nursing homes, and when those patients died, there was often no one available to pick up their bodies for days.

For those in nursing homes, all of this also spelled incredible loneliness. Residents were forced to take meals alone. Families weren't permitted to visit. Staff were overburdened and kept their distance, often reluctant to assist with bathrooming and basic personal hygiene. Over the first seven months of the pandemic, 80,000 people died in nursing homes, cut off from their families.[40]

On April 10, I appeared on Rachel Maddow's show on MSNBC to help bring some focus on this. "People over 80 today were born at or around the Great Depression. Many of them served in the Korean War. They have lived through so much in this country. And the promise that Medicare and Medicaid in our country owes to these people is a dignified life, a healthy life, and a peaceful existence to their last days. Sadly, this is not what's happening."[41]

When Dan Patrick, or Trump's White House advisor Scott Atlas, or Donald Trump himself suggested that COVID-19 is only a problem of old people, and that they should be isolated so that other Americans can get on with their lives, they were putting people in danger without giving them much say in the matter. The idea that the country could effectively isolate millions of people is a myth, and a cruel one at that. The virus spreads based on the kind of random interactions that are difficult to control. In Sweden, calls to simply isolate the elderly so that the lives of other Swedes could go on relatively normally did not, in fact, end up protecting the elderly: people age 70 and older have accounted for 88 percent of Swedish COVID-19 deaths.[42] Japan, on the other hand, reacted quickly and with uniformity. With little more than 1,000 deaths in the country as a whole, only 14 percent of those deaths were in elder-care facilities. That is compared with more than 40 percent in the United States, despite a lower proportion of U.S. seniors living in nursing homes. When there's low transmission in a community, seniors are protected.

Of course, those who call for the "forced isolation" of the elderly miss a more fundamental point. Only 6.5 percent of seniors live in congregate care settings, which means that 93.5 percent live out in the community, often in households with multiple generations.[43] In many of those situations "isolating" one person would mean isolating an entire household, frequently including people who work for a living. Arguments like this are arguments of convenience, not of logic and certainly not of principle. The head of the World Health Organization, Tedros Adhanom Ghebreyesus, said he'd heard people say it was "fine" that the elderly were dying of COVID-19 in such high numbers. His response: "No, when the elderly are dying it's not fine. It's a moral bankruptcy."[44]

There are also more people than just the elderly who live in congregate settings. On April 19, Rebecca Cokley, who is one of the country's fiercest and smartest disability advocates and who served as a deputy in both the Department of Education and the Department of Health and Human Services under Obama, sent me a plaintive and angry note about all the people she knew who were dying in nursing homes, including many of her friends and acquaintances.

"Nursing homes aren't just old people. They are forgotten people," she told me. "People like you need to do a much better job speaking up."

Her words stung. They were an assault on my self-image as someone who listened and helped. But she was right. As much as I tried to listen to Rebecca or to Dennis Heaphy, a friend and Boston-based disability advocate, I could never know what their lives were like. Meanwhile, both of them had clear visions not just of their own plight but of the plight of African Americans, of essential workers, of immigrants, of people in prison, and of Native Americans on reservations.

Dennis described the pandemic for people like him in stark terms: "This is about fighting for corporations and the economic well-being of the 1 percent at the expense of people like myself, people with disabilities, elders, African Americans. . . . [We are the] collateral damage to moving forward with such a great vision of an economy that only supports a few people."

Frontline Health Care Workers

People with the most exposure—and often the least protection—were the very people we were asking to keep us alive. An early paper in *The Lancet* showed that health care workers were three times more likely than the general population to test positive for COVID-19.[45] If the health care worker happened to be a person of color, they were five times more likely to test positive—and of course the risk of death was higher too. Even workers who had access to good PPE had a higher likelihood of testing positive than the general population, though not as high as those without adequate PPE. And people of color were less likely to be given adequate PPE by their employer.

The Guardian and Kaiser Health News built a public database of health care workers who have died in the pandemic.[46] It includes nurses (who have suffered the greatest number of fatalities), doctors, first responders, social workers, culinary and janitorial staff, administrators, and others. It also includes a short bio of each person who has died. They asked me to write a memorial tribute to those we lost. Here is an abbreviated version of what I wrote:

> They chose not to hold their own children's hands so they could hold ours. They intubated us and kept our ICU rooms germ-free. They brushed our teeth and switched our position so we could be more comfortable. As they always have, they put our health first, although this time it was in place of their own. When you enter the rooms of infected patients day in and day out with a mask that you were supposed to replace last week, your low-risk age or good health are less of a defense.
>
> The first known emergency room physician to die in the US, Frank Gabrin, sent the following text message to a friend: "Don't have any PPE that has not been used." He passed away only four days after developing symptoms, telling his husband in his final moments, "Baby, I can't breathe."
>
> As long as the patients keep coming, there will be someone to care. Let's not ask more medical professionals to pay the price they don't need to pay. They aren't just medical professionals. They are our neighbors who get the early bus, our friends who always pick up the phone, our sisters who make us laugh, our dads who always know what to say. They have their own lives and we must give them that chance.

CHAPTER 9

THE FOLLY OF THE FREE MARKET PANDEMIC

Scene: The U.S. health care system

While millions were getting infected, hundreds of thousands were dying, and millions more were losing employment, the system wasn't failing everybody. Between March and September 2020, the nation's billionaires grew $845 billion richer.[1] Capitalism, which is supposed to be an efficient way of allocating goods and services to the places of highest need, had become a perversion of itself. Shortages were everywhere, small businesses were shuttered, unemployment was high, and yet, with expenses low, companies saw soaring profits, particularly in health care.

The stock market, after an initial dip, appeared to recognize significant opportunity in the pandemic. A number of factors, including low interest rates, increased demand for some luxury items and services, and new efficiencies as companies did without labor they no longer needed, sparked tremendous gains for some. If America is good at anything, it's figuring out how to make a buck. Trump, who saw in a booming market his best chance at reelection, would take no action that would interfere with companies' ability to make money.

The health care system, filled with some of the greatest scientists and clinicians in the world, had long since become driven by and dependent on the flow of money—to the chagrin of many of those same scientists and clinicians. And during the pandemic, while doctors and nurses worked long hours, risking their lives, and scientists pulled off superhuman feats, that fixation on money didn't go away. It wasn't clear, between the dollar and the patient, which was the tail and which was the dog. Or, as the country-and-western song says, which is the windshield and which is the bug.[2]

A Nurse's Story, Part I

When Melissa was eight years old, her mother came home from work one evening accompanied by what to Melissa seemed to be a strange-looking man. He was gaunt and weak and pale, and sores dotted his face. The hospitals, the churches, and the shelters had all turned him away, her mother told her, because he was dying of AIDS. His name was Jimmy.

Despite whispers from her friends and suspicious looks from their neighbors in Yauco, Puerto Rico, where they lived, Melissa's mom, an infection control nurse, was determined to care for Jimmy. Her mother took her into the kitchen, looked Melissa in the eye, and said, "Nosotros lo cuidaremos hasta el final. Esta es ahora su casa"—*We will take care of this man till the end. This is his home now.* Melissa helped her mom dress his wounds and spoon-feed him his meals. At eight years old, she knew she'd become a nurse just like her mom.

Thirty-five years later, Melissa, now living in New Jersey with a family of her own, would carry on her mother's ethos as she confronted a new plague.

She had in fact become an infection control nurse, after working through night classes to earn her credentials, and built a career at a local dialysis center. She cared for anyone who needed her help: businesspeople, construction workers, homeless people. And she had learned to deal with indignities that sometimes confronted people of color who worked in medicine. On occasion a new doctor, mistaking her for a member of the custodial staff, would ask her to take out the trash. She had patients refuse her care because of her skin color. She never flinched. As a single mom with two kids of her own, with a small house and a mortgage, Melissa chose to focus on what she loved: serving her patients.

One Thursday in April 2020, one of her regular patients came into the center, and Melissa immediately knew something was wrong. His lungs crackled, he was sweating through his shirt, and he looked exhausted and scared. She sat with him for the four-and-a-half-hour duration of his dialysis, reassuring him and holding his hand—doing her best to protect herself with the mask she had been wearing all day.

She knew that her clinic's infection control protocol wasn't right—though the CDC guidelines called for her to have an N95 mask, the clinic's administrators assured her that surgical masks were sufficient. Of course, even those were in short supply. Each staffer was allocated only one surgical mask per day. Occasionally she would be short a mask, and she would pick one up off the floor.

After spending an uneventful weekend with her kids, she awoke on Monday to find that she couldn't smell her morning coffee.

The U.S. Bank of Health Care

Melissa wasn't just a nurse; she was also a cog in the U.S. health care system, which by 2020 wasn't primarily about nurses, wasn't about doctors, and wasn't even about patients any longer, but—as the United States' largest industry—had come to operate centrally around money. Bandages, thermometers, medicine, gowns, and healing are one part of the system, but in the part out of view of patients, the tools of the trade include secret loans, excessive markups, monopolies, abject speculation, tax schemes, debt collectors, and big corporate salaries. Dialysis itself, which is a system that keeps the kidneys functioning—largely for low-income people of color, with the use of outdated machines—made $28 billion in revenue, almost entirely from U.S. taxpayers.[3]

As personal as health care is to you, it's the biggest industry in America. We all know people who work in health care. As of 2016, health care employs 21.8 million Americans, representing 14 percent of all jobs in the United States.[4] And while nurses, therapists, and family medicine doctors earn relatively modest incomes, the top pharmaceutical, insurance, and hospital company CEOs get paid between $21 million and $58 million annually.[5]

If you zoom in on a single exam room, or witness a surgery, or see the work of someone like Melissa, you might see health care in the United States as it used to be and as it has remained in much of the world—a system whose primary purpose is to care for people. But zoom out and what you see is a large financial system, with health care thrown in on the side to keep the financial gears churning. Patients, doctors, and nurses have become the engine that keeps the money flowing through that system.

In the years when I oversaw the country's biggest health care programs for the U.S. government—and before that, when I oversaw much of the data that the health care system produces about itself—I got a bird's-eye view of the health care system, including its silos, transactions, and components. What I saw leads me to describe U.S. health care in a way that is likely different from anything you've heard before. But this explanation might make it easier to understand what you are walking into when you attempt to navigate it as a patient. It also offers an explanation of how the health care system responded when COVID-19 arrived on our shores. Here is how to understand the system, from top to bottom.

Every single year, vast amounts of money move around the health care system. In 2018, that figure was $3.6 trillion—which amounted to 17.7 percent of our gross domestic product.[6] Where does the money come from? Where does it go? Where are all the places it leaks out along the way? Why do we spend so much and yet still feel like we don't have enough to pay for what we need?

All of the money comes from three places: the taxes we pay,

our paychecks, or directly out of our pockets. On average, about $17,000 a year total is spent for each adult in the United States from these three places combined.[7]

That $17,000 spent for each of us goes into three primary connected machines. I will refer to them as the global pharmaceutical financial machine, the big medical financial machine, and the health insurance financial machine. But much of what we pay into these machines has little to do with medical care. Altogether, about $1.1 trillion—or almost one-third of the money we pay—goes for things other than our medical care.[8] There are a lot of mouths to feed. Each of the three machines has middlemen who skim money off the top, and each machine spends considerably to sustain the status quo, including on things that are only tangentially related to caring for us. And there are built-in mechanisms to ensure that whatever happens, your costs (and the revenue the health care system makes) don't come down. As I walk through how these machines work, I will give you a few examples you may not be aware of.

The Pharma Financial Machine

Large pharmaceutical companies today are giant marketing machines as much as they are developers of new medicines. Yes, some still invent drugs and have scientists, but many of the products they sell have been developed by other, smaller biotechnology companies or by universities, or are drugs the companies have had a legal monopoly on for a long time and that they raise the price of every year, or (often in the case of cancer drugs) had their development funded by either the federal government or stock market speculators. Their profits often defy gravity—going up, but rarely going down. For all this to work, there are a few important tricks of the trade.

One essential trick is to keep these legal monopolies the government grants going as long as possible. Drug companies are granted patents, or legal monopolies, which typically last 20 years.[9] If a drug goes off patent, its price can drop as much as 60–80 percent as generic competition enters the market. So companies with patents

employ massive legal teams to prevent this from happening. They are allowed to do something called "pay for delay"—that is, they pay other companies not to introduce competing drugs that would bring the price down.

So in the pharmaceutical financial machine, one company can make money by *not* producing a drug, and another company can pay to keep a monopoly so you keep paying more.

If a company doesn't want to spend the money to pay for delay, there are alternatives. Pharmaceutical company lawyers have found other techniques, like filing a series of "patent thickets" (a web of overlapping property rights designed to slow down a competitor's commercialization efforts) and secretly funding petitions from citizens to prevent competition, both of which allow them to add years to their monopolies.

Another thing that has become important in the pharmaceutical financial machine is to be able to keep raising prices every year. In most other industries, prices come down over time as competition produces newer and more efficient models. But not here. The price of thousands of drugs increases by 10 percent or more each year, and the price of a smaller group, numbering in the hundreds, increases by 100 percent or more.[10] These increases are possible only because the biggest purchaser of drugs, the federal government, is not permitted by Congress to negotiate their price. Why is that, you ask? That is the principal achievement of the most powerful lobby in Washington, D.C.: the pharmaceutical lobby.

Blocking the government's ability to negotiate drug prices is a miraculous accomplishment the drug lobby has sustained year after year and is worth untold billions. It is important not simply for the obvious reason of allowing companies to charge as high a price as they want. The other reason is it gives Wall Street unlimited opportunity to speculate in the biotech market. The research into new drugs is now frequently done by biotechnology companies that have a single drug and are often worth billions of dollars years in advance of the drug even being ready for a clinical trial. Speculators buy and sell the stock entirely based on perceptions of

how much money they think the drug will generate in the future. So when Congress gives companies unchecked pricing power, it takes the lid off how much speculators can make.[11] Indeed, sometimes great breakthrough medications or vaccines are created. But speculators and company founders can make money by selling stock even if drugs never come to fruition.

Another way drug companies maintain high prices is by paying the insurance companies a percentage of the price of a drug in the form of a rebate. The more expensive the drug, the bigger the rebate. This system is good for everybody—except the patient, that is. When it comes to prescription drug prices, Americans often pay 10 times more than Canadian or British people for a pharmaceutical product that is for all intents and purposes identical, often with the exact same formulation and sometimes made in the same factory.[12]

And while the pharma financial system eschews what it calls "government overreach" in regulating prices, it is more than happy to take more than $30 billion the taxpayers spend each year through the National Institutes of Health to do much of the research that makes these new drugs easier to discover and less risky to invest in.[13] Drug companies also take advantage of billions more in tax breaks for research and development and for drug promotion—tax breaks that they have assiduously lobbied for over the years.

It's not just what the pharma financial system does. It's what it doesn't do. Take one of our major health threats: antibiotic-resistant bacteria. As bacteria grow more resistant, we are approaching the day when people may once again die from common infections as they used to centuries ago. We have known about this threat for a long time, and yet pharmaceutical companies aren't creating new antibiotics. Why? There isn't enough financial incentive. The price of a biologic cancer drug can be 300 times the price of an antibiotic.[14] A system centered on research and cures would make different decisions than would a system focused on finance and speculation.

The pharmaceutical financial machine is so lucrative, with $1.25 trillion in revenue in 2019 industry-wide, that many others are in on the action.[15] These players include pharmacy benefit managers

who negotiate which drugs are available to you at what price, drug distributors who deliver hundreds of millions of pills, the pharmacies themselves, home infusion businesses, marketing companies, and clinical trial companies; *each* of these is a multibillion-dollar industry, and none of them makes a single medicine.

Drug companies spend far more on marketing than they spend on discovering drugs.[16] So much of the money and effort of major global pharmaceutical companies goes not only toward marketing directly to patients (those lovely TV ads) but also toward payments to doctors. Doctors are accustomed to getting stipends and expensive trips from pharmaceutical companies, but small reforms now disguise many of these payments as speaking fees, compensation for sitting on advisory boards, honoraria, and medical director fees. In 2016, drug companies spent $20 billion on marketing to those who choose what drug to give you. In fact, physicians and hospitals are legally paid $10 billion in direct fees every year from pharma companies.[17]

The Medical Financial Machine

You may view your doctor—if you are lucky enough to have one—as the person who takes care of you. Undoubtedly, that's how the doctor looks at it too. Yet the "bank of health care" sees something different when it looks at your doctor: green. Doctors can get paid by pharmaceutical companies for promoting drugs, prescribing a specific drug, or recruiting patients for clinical trials. In some specialties—especially oncology and areas such as ophthalmology—drug companies allow doctors to participate directly in the pharma financial machine by adding on to the profit margin for the drugs they provide to patients and keeping the extra for themselves. This can amount to thousands of dollars in pure profit for a doctor administering a single dose of an expensive drug.[18] One year, Melissa's employer, a national for-profit dialysis company, made 40 percent of its entire profit from just administering a single drug to its patients.

Hospitals get paid in all the same ways doctors do. Every time a drug is injected into you in a doctor's office or hospital, a bunch of money goes into the pocket of the doctor or the hospital. And the more expensive the drug they give you, the more money they pocket. Congress has allowed this to happen, again thanks to the achievements of the pharmaceutical lobby. Many members of Congress effectively get a cut of the action because pharmaceutical companies are the largest funders of political campaigns.[19]

Many of these financial opportunities exist for specialties like orthopedics, oncology, ophthalmology, cardiology, and neurology, as well as the many subspecialties within them—but not for their poorer cousins, such as family medicine, pediatrics, and mental health, and not for community clinics, emergency rooms, and other frontline areas whose goals are more preventative. The job of keeping you from getting sick is not a lucrative one. When COVID-19 began, our system was hobbled by being so heavily weighted toward these big expensive specialties, with little money for prevention and public health.

To hospitals in the medical financial system, doctors look as much like referring agents as they do healers. For a hospital, having a patient referred for a procedure or a medical stay can be incredibly lucrative. "Heads in beds" is the mantra of the medical financial system.[20] Hospitals think of your doctor the same way General Motors might think of a car dealer. That's why hospitals have been buying up physician practices—to get a lock on their patients' illnesses.

The company Melissa worked for is a prototypical part of the financial machine. Not only didn't her clinic supply sufficient PPE to her, but the company has a record of infection control violations and of paying illegal kickbacks to physicians for directing patients to them. They have settled cases for committing fraud on taxpayers, and there are numerous stories about how they have discouraged patients from taking the best medical course—like having a transplant—because it reduces the revenue from people on dialysis.

Mergers of all kinds are a big part of the medical financial system. As the number of independent hospitals has shrunk, the amount hospitals can charge has increased because they are more frequently the only game in town.[21] There are many nonprofit and religious hospitals, but the distinction between nonprofit and for-profit often has more to do with tax status and ownership than their profitability. The size, the business practices, and the executive pay can be similar. Being registered as a nonprofit or religious hospital can allow a $20–$30 billion corporation with tens of thousands of employees to pay no federal corporate or state income taxes.[22]

As in the pharmaceutical financial machine, much of the money in the medical financial machine has little to do with patient care. Some of it comes from the government for important things like cancer research or educating medical students. Some comes from donors—often prominent members of the community who may donate for a number of reasons, not least of which is to secure their *own* medical care as they age or become ill. Some payments are just giant lump sums that get sent every month by the government, subsidies that have little or nothing to do with the health care provided.

Hospitals can make a significant amount of money by lending money to the states they are located in. It works like this: States can get money from the federal government to pay for health care for the uninsured if they can put up some matching funds. For example, if a state puts up $200 million, the federal government might provide an additional $800 million in funding. Since states don't usually have $200 million lying around, they will, in effect, ask the hospitals to put up that money. The money that goes back to hospitals is not divided up based on how many uninsured patients that hospital sees. It is based on who lent the most money. Putting up a share of $200 million and getting a share of $800 million back is a pretty good deal. But it has nothing to do with caring for patients.[23]

Like the pharmaceutical machine, the medical financial machine has its own middlemen who take their bite out of the pie—technology vendors and large purchasing organizations each have their own industries worth tens of billions of dollars. Billing and collection services take a piece of the action by getting people like my friend Jeff's widow, Lynn, to pay up. Companies that make expensive MRI machines and other medical supplies and equipment—some of which works only marginally better than older technology—make billions, and spend a great deal to convince doctors that their products are superior. We need many of these services, but since such a large number of them get a piece of the action (collection services) or are used to attract patients (fancy equipment), there is often little incentive to reduce waste or lower prices—which goes toward the $17,000 we each pay. And if the price of something rises too much, a new industry will form that will sell the service of reducing that price—usually in exchange for a piece of the action.

The Insurance Financial Machine

Health insurance has become a great business. It's a business in which you can get paid to hold on to money and to keep as much of it as possible by paying for as little care—and as little *for* that care—as possible. What you pay in premiums is typically a good deal more than you receive in health care. However, there's a magical thing that happens when your employer pays money to an insurance company: they can deduct 100 percent of it from their taxes (which in 2017 amounted to $250 billion per year in taxpayer subsidies).[24] So before they've done a single thing, insurance companies' products are worth billions of dollars.

And unlike a bank, which pays *you* interest, with health insurance companies you pay *them* interest: they are required to spend only 80 percent of the money they get from you on your health care. For that money, almost all Americans are dissatisfied with insurance companies, routinely rating them in the bottom five industries.[25]

■ ■ ■

The big financial health care machines can do what they do because of the significant influence they buy in Washington, where the rules get made. I can't remember a single time when anyone in the health care system made an urgent phone call or came to see me while I was head of CMS because of something involving a patient. It was always about money. One CEO even threatened to pull out of the Affordable Care Act if we didn't help approve a highly lucrative merger he had in front of the Justice Department. We didn't help, and he kept his word to punish us, though the ones who really got punished were people who had his company's insurance and lost it.

If all Americans were getting their health care needs met, many would not object to reasonable levels of profit for the health care sector. But, for all this machinery, patient care in the United States compares very unfavorably with other countries despite being twice as expensive, and getting more expensive every year. And as the average life expectancy in this country declines, fewer Americans can afford the health care they need. And that was before the pandemic hit.

A Nurse's Story, Part 2

Melissa was running a 104-degree fever and every muscle in her body ached, even the muscles in her jaw. She knew she was fighting for her life.

A few nights into her illness, Melissa was so weak she had to get on all fours to climb up the 13 stairs to get to her bedroom, stopping to rest on each step. It felt like climbing 13 mountains. When she reached the top, she collapsed on the floor. She woke up to the sound of her son crying and screaming her name. He thought she was dying before his eyes. She begged, "No, no, please don't come near me."

Melissa knew she had no choice but to go to the hospital. She had cared for many patients at the end of their lives, so the next morning, she asked her boyfriend to collect some paperwork before she left—the deed to her house, insurance information, and child custody documentation—so that he could make arrangements more easily once she died. With little energy to speak, she called a friend who was a lawyer. She wanted to die well, on her own terms, unlike the horror she so often saw on the news.

She said goodbye to her kids, who were crying and hugging each other. She climbed into the passenger seat of her boyfriend's Honda. As he pulled out of the driveway, he patted her hand. Melissa could hear her kids sobbing inside, begging her to stay alive.

Fortunately, she didn't die, but it took 25 days before Melissa felt like she was starting to recover. Soon after, her employer started pressuring her to come in. After five hours on the job on her first day back, she passed out. When she woke up, she was in an ambulance, on the way back to the hospital.

The Pandemic Economy

The U.S. response to the pandemic differed from the response in other parts of the world largely in the degree to which the government was reluctant to interfere with our system of laissez-faire capitalism, even if it was for the public good. Given the sparseness of the U.S. public health system (outlined in Chapter 2), the frontline response was driven by the private system. Treating patients, selling tests, creating masks, and researching cures would all come from the same financially oriented system that allowed prices and profits to float freely, and for which taxpayers paid the price. Taxpayer money and scarcity-level pricing made health care stocks jump 65 percent between the latter part of March and the first part of August.[26]

The Pandemic Gold Rush: Masks

Mark Parkinson is a former governor of Kansas. Today, he's the CEO of the National Center for Assisted Living. Tens of thousands died in nursing homes in the early months of the pandemic, often when nursing home workers were forced to work without protective gear and travel from center to center, often spreading the virus. In September, I asked Mark whether assisted living centers were able to find PPE. He told me they ran so short of supplies that they routinely had to buy PPE at as much as 10 times the market rate and still never had enough.[27]

For some, seeing shortages in the U.S. health care system is like seeing a gold rush. Millions of Americans were in desperate need of medical care, clinicians needed supplies, and the country needed new drugs, vaccines, and diagnostic tests. The gold rush was made possible by both our lack of preparation in building our reserves of the basic things we need in a pandemic and the federal government's trepidation in interfering with markets. All over the country, medical facilities were in a desperate scramble for masks, and people like Melissa were told they didn't need them. By the time the United States faced the fact that the virus was coming here, global supplies were disappearing.

Kentucky governor Andy Beshear told me, "I'm not sure I can describe . . . how it felt early on. . . . Here in Kentucky, we would spend all day long, me included, on the phone trying to buy necessary PPE, not just the N95 masks. And every single rabbit hole that we ran down, you couldn't get any."[28]

To speed up delivery of PPE, the federal government eased regulations on vendor competition and provided over $1.8 billion to hundreds of unvetted contractors by the end of May alone.[29] So with skyrocketing demand, government funding, and unlimited pricing power, just about everyone from local business owners to college students jumped on the opportunity to profit, able to "arrange" purchase of cheaper pallets of masks from China and market them at exorbitant prices. To make matters worse, many of the masks being offered weren't what they claimed to be. According to Andrew Stroup at Project N95, the nonprofit venture I helped get off the ground to find masks for health care workers, in the early days 80 percent of all N95 masks being offered turned out to be counterfeit or from companies without a history of mask development.[30]

3M, the largest U.S. manufacturer of masks, claimed it had added manufacturing lines and was now producing 50 million masks a month.[31] Yet none could be found except in one place—the internet. Every day I received emails and texts with offers to sell me up to a million 3M masks, all while doctors and nurses struggled without protective gear. One morning in late March, coffee cup in hand, I decided to call 3M . I asked to speak to their CEO, Mike Roman. Moments later, I got a call back from the government affairs department.

I asked if the company was beginning to manufacture more N95 masks in the crisis. The person I spoke to said that yes, they were, and had already reached capacity. I asked how long it would take to create new capacity. I had done enough homework to know that U.S. companies making respiratory masks had been shutting down capacity for a number of years as prices declined and demand slowed. He said it wouldn't be possible to create more masks in the near term. He wasn't oozing with a sense of urgency.

In a crisis, I imagined, there were many ways to increase capacity.

"Do you have masks being sent to countries like Korea that don't have shortages?"

"Yes."

"Do you have masks going to preexisting orders with non-health-care contracts, like construction workers and painters?"

"We sell to 3M distributors and don't track where they sell them."

I got the sense that a large portion of their production could be channeled to U.S. hospitals and nursing homes if they wanted to make the effort. "Given the crisis, maybe you could redirect those to U.S. hospitals," I suggested.

He said 3M couldn't break the contracts or they would get sued.

"Let me help you with that. I'm sure we could enlist the White House to help, given the crisis," I offered.

He thought about that but seemed uneasy.

"How many additional masks would you have if you could access all of those masks?" I asked.

"We have no way of knowing. We sell to distributors. So we don't have any idea where they end up," he reiterated.

This was the likely explanation for all the 3M masks being marketed in all corners of the internet for $5 and $8 per mask, as opposed to the standard $2 per mask, and for all the emails I was receiving.[32] 3M distributors (or their customers or in-laws) were creating a black market in the product. The black market was spilling over to masks of lesser quality than the N95s. Boxes of thin surgical masks that normally cost only a couple of dollars were being sold for $50 to $100.

"So how many masks are sitting in factories or falling off wholesaler trucks and ending up in the black market?" I wondered.

"We couldn't possibly know," the 3M rep replied.

Were they not watching TV? I was betting that hundreds of millions of masks could likely be made available to hospitals if 3M cared to do something about it, such as redirect supply and shut down counterfeiters.

Unlike when I was in the government, this time I had no stick to persuade him with. "You do see all the nurses and doctors dying because they can't access your product?" I asked.

"We're doing everything in our power. We've ramped up production."

I took one more shot—one I'd never imagined I would take.

"Look, the reason I'm calling you is I think you're about to be in the barrel."

"What do you mean?" he asked.

"It's about to be your turn. I hate to see this happening to a good Minnesota company," I said.

"See *what* happening?"

"Right now the country is focused on ventilators, but you're next up. The White House is about to come after you," I suggested.

"What do you mean? How?"

"DPA for sure," I said, using the initials of the Defense Production Act, which allowed the government to direct companies
to use production capabilities to produce goods required in states
of emergency. Given how far behind the country had started out, I
believed we needed to be using this tool much more aggressively.
If I'd had anything to say about it, the DPA would have been in-
voked with mask manufacturers in January 2020. Trump had so
far refused to do it. I was about to try to get him to.

"Probably a Trump tweet as well," I added.

"Are you serious? Is there someone we can talk to in the White
House?"

"Yes, I can get you to someone on Trump's team. But if I were
you, I would have that conversation quickly. Let me talk to them,"
I said.

He thanked me, and we hung up.

I called Adam Boehler at the White House and told him everything I knew. I explained that I believed 3M could produce way more
inventory if pressure was applied, and I gave him the contact at 3M.

Naturally, I took to Twitter with what I had learned. "NOW:
Email, text, or call @3M and ask them how many of their masks
are going to US medical community or other countries with shortages vs. others? We can't needlessly lose health care workers. They
must make this public. And then change."[33]

A day after my tweet, it was reported that 280 million masks in
warehouses around the U.S. were purchased by foreign buyers—in
a single day.[34] A spokesperson for FEMA said that the agency had
not "encouraged or discouraged U.S. companies from exporting
overseas." What that meant, in essence, was that we were supporting the free market ideology—not to mention the black market—
instead of getting PPE to nurses and doctors.[35] Later we would learn
that Trump initiated a trade deal that resulted in U.S. manufacturers
sending $17.6 million worth of masks and other PPE to China in
January and February, even though he knew the virus was coming
to our shores.[36]

At the end of February, as cases began to grow in South Korea, the South Korean government took a very different approach than the U.S. government. They purchased 50 percent of all the KF94 masks (the Korean equivalent of the N95) produced by South Korean manufacturers and sold them to pharmacies, agricultural cooperatives, and post offices at $1.23 per mask.[37] These venues were allowed to sell them for only pennies higher. In early March, seeing that demand was still not being met, the government increased its share of KF94 purchases to 80 percent. By the end of March, 3M was still sending masks to Korea that Koreans didn't need, so people there were turning around and selling back into the United States for $4.50 or more.

Boehler called me later, as upset as I was. He had gotten the runaround at 3M. He was floored that they wouldn't even put their CEO on the phone with the White House.

"Ninety-nine percent of companies are great. These guys are unbelievable. So intransigent. They don't understand this is wartime. What do you think we should do?" Boehler asked.

"I completely agree. I don't think they get that people are dying. DPA them," I said. "I can't believe I'm saying this: ask the president to tweet at them."

Boehler said he would talk to Trump.

Once in a while a plan works. On April 2, Trump tweeted, "We hit 3M hard today after seeing what they were doing with their Masks. 'P Act' all the way. Big surprise to many in government as to what they were doing—will have a big price to pay!" The same day, he announced at a press conference that he would invoke the DPA (what he called the "P Act") to authorize FEMA to procure as many masks from 3M as needed.[38]

On April 6, Trump announced plans to purchase 55.5 million masks a month from 3M. The popular press reported this as a brilliant success and a patriotic move by 3M, a great American company. Trump got credit for being a great dealmaker, which I laughed about. A month later, the Department of Defense signed a $126 million contract with 3M to start producing masks in October, for a total of 312 million masks.[39]

Sadly, 312 million masks is a drop in the bucket, and production beginning in October 2020 didn't come in time for Melissa and many others. Hundreds of frontline health care workers have died because they didn't have adequate protective gear.

As of November 2020, three times more health care workers have died in the United States than the total number of people who have died in South Korea.[40]

Pandemic Profits: Pharma and Biotech

One of the greatest scientific efforts the world has ever seen began in January 2020—the race to develop a vaccine, test it out on volunteers, manufacture it, and distribute it to the public, all within 12 to 18 months. From sequencing the virus in a lab to running the clinical trials to building concurrent manufacturing capacity, the achievement was a testimony to amazing advances in science, the bravery of the trial participants, a little bit of luck . . . and a lot of money.

When Congress put in place $3 billion for vaccine research, the appropriations bill originally included a provision requiring simply "affordable pricing" for the vaccine. But the pharmaceutical lobby successfully had that provision removed. In the end, even with $1 billion worth of funding for research and a large purchase from the government, Moderna ended up selling its vaccine at about twice the cost of an influenza vaccine.[41]

The Trump administration was on the side of drug companies. Before the bill came to Congress in February, Secretary Azar was already signaling to the pharmaceutical companies that they could charge whatever they wanted for a lifesaving coronavirus vaccine. "We can't control that price because we need the private sector to invest," Azar said.[42]

Having someone pay much of your costs to develop a product and still allow you to charge as much as you want is a new definition of the phrase "never let a good crisis go to waste." (Unlike the other companies, Pfizer paid its own development costs.)

Corporate executives often take care of themselves before patients see a benefit. Between January and June, before a large-scale Phase III trial even began, Moderna's stock price tripled.[43] During this time, very little data came out on the vaccine, but the company put out flattering press releases, and its CEO, Stéphane Bancel, appeared frequently on CNBC to tout the company's coming vaccine. (He turned out to be right.) As the company's stock price shot up, Bancel sold 72,000 shares of his own stock, and other Moderna executives sold stock as well.[44] Speculation in drug stocks allowed people to make money before any product was actually made. Later, in October, the company did take a step in the right direction, announcing that it would not sue anyone for violating its patents for its vaccine candidate.[45] They should be applauded for that. When Pfizer made the announcement showing its first Phase III trial data, it was an exciting day for the world of science. The scientists at BioNTech, the German firm Pfizer had partnered with, had done remarkable work. Pfizer's stock price soared. That day, Pfizer's CEO, Albert Bourla, sold $5.6 million worth of stock.

Lab testing companies, so critical to helping control the virus, saw the pandemic as their opportunity to push through reforms they felt had long been needed. In early March, I had begun calling commercial labs and asking them how quickly they could produce more tests and what needed to happen for that to work. They had a laundry list of things they wanted, but the main thing was to get paid more. They wanted the price Medicare pays for a diagnostic test to double, from the previous $51 to $100.[46]

In June, I had the opportunity to work with the NBA and Yale University on a simple test that used saliva. Spurred by the vision of Dr. Robby Sikka, the vice president of basketball performance and technology for the Minnesota Timberwolves, the project aimed to produce an open-source test that could be made and sold for as low as $2 each.

In September 2020, a new antigen test came on the market that was inexpensive to produce, offering the potential to revolutionize the testing process—making it easier to test regularly and obtain results quickly. But companies were charging $150 for it. As Rockefeller Foundation president Rajiv Shah told me in October, "There's the real cost and what people are charging. And I think the real cost probably should be down to 30 bucks a test on the high end in just a couple of months. . . . I can tell you anecdotes of north of $200 to get a quick-result test. And this is the one area where we should be deploying these things in a way to generate public health outcomes, not maximize profits."[47]

I asked Mark Cuban what he thought the obligation of a company to its shareholders is during a crisis. His answer: "To keep them alive. If people die, there is no company."

The Pandemic Windfall: The Insurers

No one made more money for doing less during the pandemic than insurance companies. Americans paid tens of billions of dollars in insurance premiums during the pandemic to cover their medical care. However, fear of infection and the temporary suspension of elective procedures meant that unless you were one of the unlucky ones with COVID-19, you weren't going to the doctor or getting treatment. So what happened to all that money we handed to insurance companies to pay for those medical costs? They kept it, of course, as profits. Even as 7.7 million people lost insurance from their employers, four insurance companies made nearly $14 billion in profits between April and June 2020 alone. As Americans were dying and getting sicker and sicker, the largest health insurers saw their profits literally double from April through June.[48]

Insurance without losses is a great business. But it might tell us something about the system we have set up.

The Pandemic Industry

While other countries were busy wrestling the pandemic under control, the pandemic industry itself became a multibillion-dollar business in the United States, with lots of government funding, money being passed out quickly, and companies focused on churning out profits.

Corporations all over the country were filing to receive loans designed for small businesses, and something of a cottage industry broke out to get the Treasury Department to change the rules so that private-equity-backed companies and large corporations could get a portion of that money, including $18.3 million to firms linked to Trump himself.[49] Small companies with no banking relationships could not exert such influence and most were not able to secure loans. And, of course, the businesses that were used to the way things worked in Washington had lobbyists file their paperwork on the first day, since they knew the government funds allocated to this program would soon run out. People like former New Jersey governor and Trump associate Chris Christie got paid hundreds of thousands of dollars lobbying to get extra money for businesses.[50]

While Americans died in record numbers, people couldn't get test results for a week or more, nurses and doctors went without masks, and small physician-run clinics shuttered, business was still booming for big health. Whether you believe capitalism has some role to play in health care or not, during the pandemic the system only served its masters. The total revenue of the 30 largest U.S. pharmaceutical companies, insurance companies, for-profit hospitals, and medical device companies in the second quarter of 2020 was $467 billion.[51] If you expected a global pandemic with thousands of Americans dying each day to challenge that, you didn't understand the U.S. system.

A Nurse's Story, Part 3

If the crisis revealed how our health care system worked, it also revealed how much the people in it—the people we call heroes—really matter. By the end of June, Melissa had "recovered," but like many people who came down with COVID-19, she had residual symptoms. There was pain in her left arm from shoulder to fingertips— sometimes at night it was so intense that it woke her up. She had her appetite back but still sometimes got frequent and intense bouts of nausea and diarrhea. If she went out for three hours, she needed to sleep for 12.

But that wasn't where her problems ended. She wasn't yet able to go back to work, so she wasn't getting paid by the dialysis company. She applied for unemployment benefits but was denied because technically she was still employed. She had been loyal to the company she worked for and had thought they were loyal to her, but now that she was sick, she realized she was as disposable as the surgical masks she'd had to hunt for on the floor. Melissa felt something many of us have—that we are no longer the focus of the health care system, but an afterthought in a system that's lost sight of why it exists in the first place.

CHAPTER 10

ANTI-EXPERT, PRO-MAGIC

Scene: The world of science and doubters

> Preparation was our first chance. When that failed, a national strategy was our next option. When that failed, a humane and unified approach was our next option. If all we have left are miracle cures, that's a nation that needs to look itself in the mirror.
>
> —Andy Slavitt in *Mother Jones*, September 19, 2020[1]

In New Zealand, the first sign of a cluster of cases resulted in strict orders to stay at home, halting any outbreak in its tracks. In the United States, the fundamental elements of reducing the spread, and with it the illnesses and deaths from the virus, seemed uniquely out of reach. With cooperation, sustained behavior change, and political leadership all seemingly off the table, the United States was pinning its hopes on a single poorly understood thing: a vaccine.

Vaccines

Nothing symbolized America's love-hate relationship with science and expertise more than vaccines.

Vaccines may be one of the world's greatest inventions. Prior to the vaccine being introduced for measles in 1963, 2.6 million children worldwide died every year from what in 2020 feels entirely preventable. Yet in recent years, in the United States, as in France, Canada, Austria, and other wealthy countries, there has been a growing distrust of vaccines. Luxuriously removed from the hardships of a life without the advances of science, living high atop the world's hierarchy, Americans left as many as 2 percent of kindergartners (more than 100,000 children) unvaccinated as of 2018. If this were only a personal choice—an individual liberty—no one would care very much. But if enough people are left unvaccinated, every case of measles gets spread to 12 to 18 other people. Cases multiply quickly, and deaths follow. And, of course, children don't exactly have a say in whether they're vaccinated.[2]

The promise of a vaccine for COVID-19 has been a key part of the strange theater of our pandemic response. When the administration talked about science, it was not presented as something to be respected as much as it was a way to promise results without doing the harder work. That work, guided by science, would have included a national testing and contact tracing strategy, a mask mandate, and in areas with high infection rates temporarily closing indoor places that attract crowds. All those things in combination with a vaccine were the recommended scientific approach—and would have saved a lot of lives. But unlike those other interventions, when it came to a vaccine, no one in the general public needed to lift a finger.

As early as February 2020, Trump began promising a vaccine would be coming soon (in fact, large-scale clinical trials didn't begin until September).[3] Trump and Pence were busy selling units in a condo that hadn't been built yet. Pence published an op-ed in the *Wall Street Journal* on June 16, before cases started to rise dramatically in the southern part of the United States, saying, "We've slowed the spread, we've cared for the most vulnerable, we've saved lives, and we've created a solid foundation for whatever challenges we may face in the future. That's a cause for celebration, not the media's fear mongering." But when that turned out not to be the case, Pence suggested on August 21 that there would be "a miracle around the corner," in reference to a vaccine.[4] In reality, vaccines normally take years to be developed, proven safe and effective, and distributed, and even an accelerated timeline would mean vaccines wouldn't reach the general public until 2021.

For an administration that stymied and belittled its scientists at every turn, that was a lot of confidence to place in science. Pence couldn't even use the word *science* or *scientist*, instead preferring to refer to the work that people train for and study for, and the progress achieved by experimentation and analysis, as *a miracle*. Pence's particular history with science includes the time when, as governor of Indiana, he prolonged and worsened an HIV outbreak by opposing needle exchanges; the time when he asserted that smoking cigarettes does not in fact kill; and the time he claimed condoms do not prevent sexually transmitted diseases. And, of course, Pence does not believe in climate change.[5]

When I spoke to Ed Yong, science writer for *The Atlantic*, in September 2020, we discussed the magical thinking underlying the public perception of a COVID-19 vaccine. He told me, "We are going from one silver bullet countermeasure to the next."[6] This sense that one thing could rescue us felt like a first-world way of thinking, akin to the way our disbelief that the virus could come to our shores kept us from reacting quickly enough at the start.

The truth is that our hopes in science can be as misplaced as our criticism of it. Vaccine candidates were indeed abundant, but, by themselves, vaccines cannot eradicate the virus, only slow down its spread so fewer people get deathly ill. How long a vaccine offers protection and the type of protection it offers—does it prevent infections, or does it only reduce symptoms? Does it also reduce contagiousness? Does it work in severe cases? Does it work in the elderly?—are questions science can't answer until the vaccine has been tested on enough people. This means that while vaccination in sufficient volumes would reduce the rate of transmission, it would not be enough to completely eliminate the need for mask use and other safety measures in the short run. So a vaccine is a big part of the answer, but not the answer.

Vaccines can't escape the same forces that make it difficult to fight COVID-19 through other means, such as mask wearing. Just as we all count on each other to wear masks, we all count on each other to be vaccinated. As with mask wearing, if you were the only person in your community to be vaccinated, there's a good chance it would protect you and limit your capacity to pass the virus to others, but that wouldn't do much good if the goal was to end the pandemic. Herd immunity—or stopping the spread of the virus because enough people are immune—without mass infections is the real goal of the vaccine.

A vaccine that is 100 percent effective if taken by only 50 percent of the public, is no better than a vaccine that is 50 percent effective and taken by 100 percent of the public. The goal of a vaccine is that it gets Zach's math to work in reverse and allows people to get back to pre-COVID-19 levels of interaction with only minor outbreaks from time to time. The higher the percentage of people who take it, the more quickly the virus becomes increasingly rare. So public trust is just as important as the vaccine itself.

Undermining the FDA

Even as Trump was busy promising a vaccine would arrive before the presidential election, he was simultaneously undermining the public's trust in the scientists, medical professionals, and institutions that create vaccines—a trust that had already become increasingly precarious. The length of a vaccine clinical trial cannot be dictated in advance any more than one can demand that a blizzard deliver 12 feet of snow to Minneapolis. Testing the efficacy of a vaccine requires that you give it to tens of thousands of people in a clinical trial and hope that enough of them are subsequently exposed to the virus. This group then has to be compared with a like population of people with similar exposure who received a placebo or a non-COVID-19 vaccine (for example, the meningococcal vaccine, which is the control in many of the European studies). Then the FDA has to review the results to determine whether the vaccine is effective and safe. During an emergency, those standards can become considerably less stringent, and that has been the case with COVID-19. But the standards are still rigorous—or at least they're supposed to be. However, Trump attempted to interfere in this process from the White House, undermining the trust needed in order to get people to agree to take the vaccine in the first place.[7]

Peter Marks foresaw how important public trust would be, and that drove him to exit the Operation Warp Speed effort that was his brainchild and head back to the FDA just a few days after arriving at the White House in April 2020. When Marks saw the political pressure being placed on the FDA to roll out a vaccine before the election, presumably to enhance the president's chances of being reelected, he made a monumental decision. On a mid-August phone call with members of an NIH-organized vaccine working group that included a large number of pharma execs, academics, and others not in government, he let it be known that if the FDA was overruled and a vaccine was approved before it was properly determined to be safe and effective, he would publicly resign.

"I could not stand by and see something that was unsafe or ineffective that was being put through," Marks told a reporter from Reuters. "You have to know where your red line is, and that is my red line. I would feel obliged to resign and in doing so, I would indicate to the American public that there's something wrong."[8]

Marks's message was intended for the public. But it also served to trap the president into letting the FDA do its job. And that message may have gotten there just in time. After spending three and a half years demonizing the FDA as part of the "deep state," Trump was able to bend the FDA to his will left and right by the time COVID-19 hit. His most effective method was to fire and ostracize dissenters. The attack on Nancy Messonnier for warning the American public about the coming of the pandemic after Trump and Azar had been aware of it for nearly two months was the first shot across the bow. In April, it was Rick Bright's turn. Bright, the man whose forethought allowed vaccine development to begin in early January, was demoted for, among other things, speaking out about the administration's lack of a swift response to the pandemic. Trump referred to him as "disgruntled." All of this made it easier for Trump to strong-arm the FDA into approving medications and tests with little fear of people speaking out.[9]

One of the most senior career civil servants at the FDA told me, "When the civil service staff saw what was happening [with Bright and Messonnier], it made it much more unlikely and scarier for people to speak their minds."

While he was waiting for his miracle vaccine, Trump occasionally seized on other supposed miracles, most famously with hydroxychloroquine, which in March he began to tout for its curative properties. People in the FDA could count the days from when Trump would get a call from Fox host Laura Ingraham or see a tweet from Elon Musk to when he would hold a press conference at which he'd demand that the FDA take action.[10] Soon he and Azar were pushing the FDA to grant emergency approval for hydroxychloroquine, which it did on March 28. The scientists who wrote the approval included language that, to the trained eye, signaled their deep doubts about this miracle cure. Bright objected to this in what became the last straw for Azar and Trump. But the drug was approved nonetheless, and the immediate effect was to validate Trump's promotion of an unsafe drug that was in limited supply and was needed for people with lupus. The longer-term effect was even more damaging: further undermining people's trust in scientists by allowing the public to see how easily Trump could manipulate them. As Bright said, "In this administration, the work of scientists is ignored or denigrated to meet political goals and advance President Trump's reelection aspirations."[11] In undermining the FDA's authority, Trump signaled a return to the only other alternative—the days of traveling peddlers of potions, when everyone picks their own authority.[12]

And Trump was just getting started. In August, when the FDA didn't see sufficient data to approve an age-old therapy called convalescent plasma, in which blood from a previously infected person is given to a newly infected person, he said at a news conference, "It could be a political decision because you have a lot of people over there that don't want to rush things because they want to do it after November 3."

In case it wasn't clear, Trump showed the FDA commissioner what the game was—he sent out a threatening tweet saying, "The deep state, or whoever, over at the FDA is making it very difficult for drug companies. . . . Obviously, they are hoping to delay the answer until after November 3rd." The day after the tweet, the FDA reversed course. Not only did it force approval of the therapy, but FDA commissioner Stephen Hahn held a briefing with the president in which Hahn grossly exaggerated the success of the treatment: "Many of you know I was a cancer doctor before I became FDA commissioner. And a 35 percent improvement in survival is a pretty substantial clinical benefit. What that means is—and if the data continue to pan out—100 people who are sick with covid-19, 35 would have been saved because of the admission of plasma."[13]

Unfortunately, it was not true that 35 out of 100 people with COVID-19 who were given convalescent plasma survived. In fact, *five* out of 100 survived *for a week longer*.[14] Hahn suffered the fate of many who were getting their first exposure to the president and his strong personality: he was doing his best to please Trump. And to do that, Hahn misinformed the American public on behalf of his boss.

I responded in an op-ed on NBC.com:

If you walked into the FDA tomorrow and claimed a miracle cure that could save 35 percent of those infected with COVID-19, the first thing they would do is examine those claims rigorously.

Validating claims of effectiveness is one of the most important and painstaking of the FDA's jobs. If those claims turned out to be false, the FDA would come down hard and the company could face massive civil and criminal liability.[15]

On September 23, Brodie dutifully followed me down the stairs at 10:30 p.m., as was his custom when I had a late night or early morning TV appearance. If he had been sleeping, he would rouse himself from the corner of our bedroom, follow me downstairs to my office, curl his body on top of my feet, and fall back asleep. We had done it dozens of times in the first few months of the pandemic: Brodie under the desk, me staring into the camera on my laptop. This time it was for Don Lemon's show *CNN Tonight*.

"Andy, you called it last night," Lemon said during a commercial break.

I had been on his show the night before as well, discussing FDA independence, and I'd said, "The president, as much as he would like to, can't just order people [in the vaccine trial] to have enough exposure [to COVID-19]. It will take as long as it takes, the FDA has got to do its job." But I had closed my appearance with this reminder: "Despite what the FDA said, Trump has the authority to overrule them. And don't think that that's not a possibility."[16]

The next day Trump did something close to what I had warned about. Asked by a reporter whether he was okay with the FDA considering stricter guidelines for the emergency approval of a vaccine, he said, "We may or may not approve it. That sounds like a political move, because when you have Pfizer, Johnson & Johnson, Moderna, these great companies coming up with the vaccines, and they've done testing and everything else, I'm saying, 'Why would they have to be, you know, adding great length to the process?'"[17]

The reason this protection is so crucial during a vaccine trial was summarized in an open letter to Hahn signed by hundreds of scientists: "To maximize the use of a COVID-19 vaccine(s) by the American people, it is therefore essential that the science and public health communities work with the federal government to increase public confidence in any approved or authorized product. . . . For that to happen, we must be able to witness a transparent and rigorous FDA approval process that is devoid of political considerations."[18]

In other words, politicians should stay out of it.

The incident with convalescent plasma was a turning point for Hahn. Stung by that letter and the public rebuke, Hahn issued a mea culpa on Twitter and reversed course. With newfound courage, he began to defy Trump and Azar by beginning to aggressively and publicly push back on the idea of approving a vaccine prematurely. He supported Peter Marks on releasing stricter standards for vaccine approval. There's nothing worse for a bully than when the bullied have decided they've had enough. Azar considered firing him, but he couldn't for the same reason Trump didn't fire him: it was too close to the election.[19] Instead he took the unusual step of removing Hahn's regulatory authority.[20] Trump's and Azar's core problem became that the scientific reputation of people like Hahn was now more important to them than their political one. Peter Marks and the scientists had won this one important battle.

Undermining the CDC

When it comes to deadly infectious diseases, before a vaccine is approved—and even for some time afterward—the CDC controls the most important medicine we have: public messaging. In the case of COVID-19, helping people to understand why it's in everyone's interest to practice social distancing and wear masks required consistency and persuasion. And no institution was better suited to perform those tasks than the Centers for Disease Control and Prevention.

But controlling the message was Trump's domain. Particularly

as the election grew closer, he saw the CDC as a threat to undermine his narrative that COVID-19 was well under control. A massive agency of scientists, each of whom saw what was happening
and felt they had an obligation to alert the public—as Nancy Messonnier had—was his worst nightmare. As mentioned in Chapter
2, Trump increased the number of political appointees at the CDC
from one—the director—to five. Their job was not to facilitate the
work of the career scientists on staff there but to ensure that their
work only shed a positive light on the president. As far as the president was concerned, the scientists hadn't been elected to anything,
but he had.

Part of the CDC's job in a public health crisis is to issue guidance on how schools, offices, and public places can open most safely.
Frequently, though, that guidance was altered by Trump officials to
make everything appear safer than it was. The background of those
Trump officials was not in science but in public relations. One of
them, Michael Caputo, a Trump communications aide installed at
HHS, made it his task to question the science of the CDC in order
to avert any political damage to Trump. Even innocuous but essential guidance on school protocols were reviewed by Ivanka Trump,
because it became viewed as a threat to Trump's narrative. So when
the CDC wrote anything about the virus that raised a specter of
concern, Trump's political team was there to intercept it.[21] If the
scientists managed to get it out without White House notice, they
would soon be forced to issue an embarrassing correction. Birx,
who was herself reading all of the primary studies, was incensed at
the interference. People who didn't know what they were talking
about were suppressing guidance to the public.

Apolitical institutions such as the Federal Reserve, the EPA, and
the CDC act as an important check on politics during challenging
times. These institutions had become the envy of the world over
many years, attracting talent from across the globe and investing in
research to steady the economy, improve the environment, and prevent disease. The culture of the CDC, based away from Washington
in Atlanta, was intended to be free of too much political interference.

Americans have legitimate beefs with the CDC's COVID-19 response that can't all be blamed on the president. Not only had the CDC failed to get functioning tests out as the coronavirus came to our shores, but it was slow to provide an understanding of how the virus spread, which other agencies such as FEMA needed to do their jobs. Hence the necessity for people like Blythe Adamson.

Still, the CDC had been hobbled by Trump long before the first known case of the virus. As discussed in Chapter 2, Trump made draconian cuts to the CDC's offices in other countries, including China. The purpose of these offices is to gather intelligence about diseases in real time, and in this role they are vital to our national security. Trump saw it differently: "I'm a business person. I don't like having thousands of people around when you don't need them."[22]

This dovetailed with a core mantra of Trump's: that experts aren't to be trusted. Like many of Trump's rallying cries, he didn't invent it, but he magnified a preexisting cultural shift.

"The experts are terrible. Look at the mess we're in with all these experts we have," Trump had said while on the campaign trail in April 2016, referring to U.S. foreign policy in the Middle East.[23] "I know more about ISIS than the generals do," he'd said in November 2015. And "I know more about renewables than any human being on earth," in April 2016.[24] When you know more than anyone else about foreign policy, warfare, energy, vaccines— you name it—why do you need a group of experts sitting around dreaming up regulations to make vaccines safe, or bloating your budget by learning about infections in China?

Trump also had a businessman's distaste for regulations, but not the discerning eye to distinguish a needed regulation from an unnecessary one, or the expertise around him to understand what risks he would expose the country to by eliminating the important ones. So CDC guidelines became polluted with Trump's personal politics. And our best medicine became watered down—or, worse, laced with poison. When the CDC said on August 30 that only 6 percent of the people who died from COVID-19 had actually died from the disease, because they also had other conditions,

Trump was, in effect, telling Americans to let their guard down. As I wrote on Twitter: "This political spin doesn't prevent disease. It causes it."[25]

"We've all gone [to the CDC] at one time or another believing that that was the center of such integrity and great science. And still has phenomenal scientists and great integrity. I believe it's being suppressed," Larry Brilliant said to me from his home in northern California. "[Same with] the FDA, which at one time we could be really sure that if you got FDA approval, it was like pulling teeth to get it. We've lost these two great arms of our scientific response, and our political response has been abysmal, historically bad."[26]

Being able to put out only what Trump approved, the CDC was not only imperiling the United States' ability to control the virus but also damaging its own reputation in the mind of the public. For Trump, causing doubt about the credibility of these institutions was a double win: he got his message out, and he undermined—potentially for years to come—the institutional dragons he'd come to slay.

The Scientific Process Up Close

Larry Brilliant understood the crucial role of independent experts and institutions communicating accurate information clearly during a pandemic. Under the direction of George W. Bush and his HHS secretary, Mike Leavitt, Brilliant had chaired the National Biosur-veillance Advisory Committee, created in 2004 with the purpose of preparing the country for a pandemic. His role there, and before that in eradicating smallpox, had made him widely considered one of the world's leading experts on pandemics. I spoke to him in July about how scientific experts could maintain public confidence at a time when they themselves were scrambling to learn how the virus spread.

"I think for the public as a whole," I began, "it's got to be quite maddening because to be in the middle of a scientific process, when you're not a scientist, and you hear something in January, and you hear something that's to the contrary in March, and to the contrary in April, you may not realize that that's exactly what's supposed to happen, that we are dealing with the best information we have at the time."[27]

He replied, "Well, let me agree with you that being in the middle of science is messy. It is the reason peer review is so important. And it's a reason why science has adopted a radical transparency, medical transparency approach to the way that scientists freely share information and make everything public, and print as much as possible. And that's the key, because this is a novel disease. That means nobody's ever seen it before."

But, Brilliant told me, the public continued to get the signals wrong. It could easily seem to people that our experts were constantly equivocating, when in fact they were adapting to new information as it came in: no masks, masks; transmission via surfaces, no transmission via surfaces; maintaining six feet of distance is most important, ensuring good ventilation is most important. But rather than work with the scientists to explain to the public that all they could do was offer the best information they had at the time, Trump used their uncertainty to undermine public confidence in them. Seeing the process of science taking place in real time in front of them gave some people the excuse they were looking for to not follow what public health officials were telling them. This is where Trump's undermining of science became especially dangerous.

Larry believed in "radical transparency." I considered that to extend not just to what we knew but also to how much confidence we had in what we knew, what our source was for that knowledge, and how much of that knowledge was subject to change.

Others had a similar view. Leana Wen, an emergency physician and a former health commissioner for the city of Baltimore, reiterated that much of what frustrates us about scientists is in fact a sign that they are doing their job well. "Constant reevaluation is good," she emphasized. "That's the bedrock of a strong public health response. . . . Just because it seems like our approach is changing, it doesn't mean that we are inconsistent or don't know what we're doing. In a crisis, in an emergency, you're not going to know the perfect way to do things. I think a lot of us forget that we didn't even know about this [at the beginning of 2020], that this is something that's new to the world. . . . I think that constant change is what is to be expected in this outbreak."[28]

One lesson that must be learned from our experience with COVID-19 is something Baruch Fischhoff had taught me: "If things go badly, people will overestimate how foolish the decision was. If things go well, people will underestimate its wisdom."

■■■

It's difficult to look into the future to see what we don't know today. We can, however, look at the past and see what we didn't know.

Mark Smith was one of the first physicians to treat AIDS patients in 1983 at San Francisco General Hospital.[29] In early May I called him up to get a feel for how long it had taken him and his colleagues after they saw the first AIDS patients to understand what was happening.

"It was apparent pretty quickly what we were looking at," he told me.

"How quickly?" I asked. Textbooks from that era pointed to genetics as a likely risk factor for AIDS.[30]

"Within a year or two."

At the time we spoke, the COVID-19 pandemic wasn't yet six months old.

Viewed this way, Deborah Birx's misjudgment over the summer could be seen in a more charitable way. Birx was making battlefield calls while attempting to manage the ego and politics of a president who wanted no part of the crisis. The president would have never accepted another answer.

Scientists aren't perfect, but what they have is a structure for learning, in the form of published research from around the world. By the fall of 2020, our knowledge of the virus had come a long way. We knew the places it liked to spread. We had begun to understand the importance of ventilation and air circulation. We knew which activities were relatively dangerous and which were safer, about how to test, trace, and isolate. And we knew none of these measures was impossible to implement, since we saw it being done all over the world.

Thomas Watson Jr., president of IBM from 1952 to 1971, said, "The fastest way to succeed is to double your failure rate."[31] Indeed, there are many aphorisms about failure being a natural part of science. Watching science learn about the virus and how to control it was something like watching Newton toss an apple up in the air, kick it, step on it, and throw it sideways before another apple dropped from the tree onto his head. If you came upon Newton staring at an apple hanging from the tree, and if you listened to him run all his theories by you, you might conclude he was a dummy. And if when the apple fell he offered an explanation that involved gravity, you would conclude that it had been obvious all along.

Politicians often tell you what you want to hear. Scientists can be expected to tell you the best knowledge they have at the time. And the best ones remind us of how little we know.

In the case of COVID-19, the public's difficulty in understanding what science can and cannot do was exacerbated by the fact that the virus is highly complex, so it was difficult to draw hard-and-fast conclusions.[32] As Ed Yong observed, "The thing that I keep coming back to is, this is an incredibly complex problem with lots of things that go into it."

"Including randomness, right?" I said.

"Yes! . . . Let's say state X did not do the things that everyone else did and seems to not have a high spike in cases. Therefore, [people assume] all those things that everyone else did were wrong. . . . That has been a common line of thinking. [What people often don't realize is that] stuff that happens at the far ends of the probability distribution will actually happen [some of the time]. Sometimes people will get very unlucky. Or sometimes people get very lucky. They'll get by even though they've done none of the things that will keep them safe."

Given the ambiguity, the public had the opportunity to shop for the opinions they liked the best. It is remarkable that when the Mike Osterholms of the world—who, as you will remember from Chapter 1, had been warning about a pandemic for years, only to be told that he was wrong, merely a fearmonger—were finally proven correct, even as the death count grew, "You are wrong" turned quickly into "You are exaggerating." There was always a different way to view the data if you chose. Always some comparison you could dream up. And social media birthed many experts with many ways of looking at things.

The Anti-Expert and the Pseudo-Expert

Bad faith and politics didn't help.

"A lot of people have used the fact that we are learning in real time, and there are things we don't know, and there are things that experts have gotten wrong, as this really bad-faith wedge. . . . You have this entire world of COVID truthers and contrarians and cranks," Chris Hayes, the MSNBC news personality, observed to me on a call in May.[33]

If scientists were wrong about some things, this not only invalidated their opinion, but it also promoted everyone else's. Theories and agendas pervaded social media and blogs. In the absence of knowing exactly how the virus worked, on the internet everyone's theory had equal weight.

On August 8, I wrote about the corollary to finding fault with experts—the elevation of the non-expert:

> It's not just that we have a distrust of experts, it's also that the people who dismiss experts think they're experts themselves. I find myself needing to check credentials even more closely. We have data scientists opining about T-cell immunity. We have

political advisors making proclamations about school safety. We have people who haven't taken a science class in 40 years recommending specific drugs. We have former newspaper reporters explaining epidemiology and the natural history of disease. We have legislators opining about how masks don't work. We have family doctors on Fox who consider COVID the flu. As long as things are as uncertain as they are with a novel virus, it's a chance for everybody to weigh in with their opinions.[34]

Amateurs (and the Trump administration) were all over Twitter with dangerous theories, such as encouraging individual people to purposely get infected as a step toward achieving herd immunity in the society at large. Most of the people suggesting this were not immunologists, who had an understanding of how long people might be immune, or epidemiologists, who had insight into how the virus would spread and how many would die. Rather, they were people like Dan Patrick, whose views grew out of their ideology. Occasionally non-experts got something right, and that buoyed their confidence and that of their believers. But it was like 100,000 people calling a sequence of coin flips in advance. The people who hit heads a few times in a row acted as if they were oracles—the very definition of the hindsight bias Baruch Fischhoff pointed to. Scientists such as Fauci, Frieden, Osterholm, and Brilliant, who were more cautious about reaching definitive conclusions, were discounted.

In a *USA Today* column, U.S. trade representative Peter Navarro wrote that he didn't listen to Anthony Fauci, pointing out occasions when Fauci had been wrong. In Navarro's telling, he himself had been right every step of the way and therefore was more of an expert than Fauci.[35]

Fauci was also attacked in a congressional hearing by Congressman Jim Jordan. When Fauci said he wouldn't opine on whether the government should limit protests if they might cause the virus to spread, Jordan bellowed, "You've opined on a lot of things, Dr. Fauci," and then proceeded to tell Fauci how outdoor transmission works.[36]

Part of the problem with non-experts offering their opinion is that they don't know how much is not knowable. Tom Frieden, the former head of the CDC, pointed out that on less well-understood topics, the people with the most confidence were often those who knew the least. "Within science generally, the more controversy there is, the more uncertainty there actually is. . . . Not all voices have the same credibility or validity when it comes to scientific information."[37]

But there was more than just haphazard denialism or a lack of scientific understanding at work; there was also a cynical media manipulation strategy by the White House and its allies, crafted in response to the many actual experts crying out that the president's policies, or lack thereof, were hurting and even killing people.

The administration knew the virus was worse than they let on. At the end of August, the House Select Subcommittee on the Coronavirus Crisis revealed that since June it had been receiving private reports directly from the White House Task Force saying over and over that the virus was getting worse in many states.[38] The states were also receiving these reports. Meanwhile, the first of these, which went to the subcommittee on June 23, 2020, put seven states in the "red zone," with case increases ranging from 70 percent (Arizona) to 87 percent (Florida) to 134 percent (Idaho). This was one week after Pence published his op-ed titled "There Isn't a Coronavirus 'Second Wave.'" The report on July 5—again, coming from the team inside the White House—said 15 states were now in the red zone. Two days later, Trump said, "I think we are going to be in two, three, four weeks, by the time we next speak, I think we're going to be in very good shape."[39]

The scientists in the White House presented their data, the president contradicted it, and governors in the most endangered states sided with the president. As I wrote in early August, "When all opinions are equal, hierarchy decides right from wrong."[40]

Scientists became disposable as soon as they disagreed with Trump. As data from the summer showed Birx that the virus was in fact not on its way to being handled and that the IHME's initial estimate of deaths was sadly too low, she grew concerned and announced that the virus is "extraordinarily widespread." Trump attacked Birx and soon appointed Scott Atlas as his White House scientific advisor.[41]

Scott Atlas was Trump's new expert. He had caught Trump's attention on Fox News offering exactly the opinion the president sought—there was nothing to be done about COVID-19, and in any case it wasn't very harmful to most people. Atlas, a former professor of radiology at Stanford, had no training in infectious diseases, virology, or epidemiology. But he denounced the resistance to unsafe school openings as "hysteria," pushed for the resumption of college sports, and blamed the infection spike in southern states on protests and border crossers. He supported Trump's penchant for inaction by pushing theories of herd immunity that would have resulted in hundreds of thousands of needless additional deaths and gave the administration cover to say that they had scientific support.[42] Upon Atlas's arrival, Birx no longer had access to the president.[43] The scientific community, and even Atlas's colleagues at Stanford, raised the alarm.[44]

Atlas's appointment fulfilled a prophecy I had made back in May when Trump was pressing to open the country and ignoring public health measures. I had written, "Now expect to hear more from 'counter-scientists,' discrediting the 'doom and gloom' people who want to keep the economy down. Anyone with halfway decent credentials, who is willing to say that economies should open now, will have an opportunity to make a new career as a cable pundit."[45]

But my prediction wasn't magical. I had participated in a phone call in May with Reince Priebus, Trump's first (and long since exiled) chief of staff. Priebus had been discussing political strategy at a time when the scientific community was urgently warning about the dangers of COVID-19. He had been in the White House recently and recalled that their goal was to find an expert they could put up against the hundreds who were on TV giving messages contrary to the White House's wishes. Even one expert offering a contrary opinion plays into cable TV's penchant for presenting both sides of any issue and would allow Trump to assert that a largely settled issue was a matter of dispute among experts. Atlas's choice as the most important scientific advisor to the president, without a single infectious disease credential, was a statement on where the country stood on placing value on expertise.

Why wouldn't we follow the lead of other countries that had found some success? Here we were, pandemic novices. While the United States had been badly behind South Korea at the start, over time it had become clear that the approach the East Asian countries were taking was working, while ours wasn't. It was one thing to start off badly, but why didn't we adapt?

Scott Atlas may be the perfect metaphor. We wouldn't follow any other country's example because, like Atlas, we were novices who considered ourselves experts.

This is part and parcel of the feeling of American exceptionalism. The United States doesn't have the humility to follow. We think we must always lead. We keep telling ourselves we're the best even when evidence suggests we are not. Our mentality suggests we would rather risk being last than come in second or third.

By fall, COVID-19 cases in the United States began a climb to record numbers, and with those increased cases came more hospitalizations and more deaths. During the second wave, once again, the United States led the world in cases and deaths. But scientific failure wasn't to blame. Ultimately, the failure of the U.S. government to protect its citizens—and our failure to protect each other—was a failure not of our expertise but of our cultural attitude toward expertise. Our most dangerous enemy—aided and abetted by the president—turned out to be not the virus itself but our own willingness to distort reality and turn our backs on one another. Our ability to successfully face future crises will depend a great deal on how well we can turn that around—on our willingness to trust experts, trust each other, and see things as they are.

CHAPTER 11

DENIERS, FAUXERS, AND HERDERS (OH MY)

SCENE: CABLE TV AND SOCIAL MEDIA

"On March 14, to name one among countless possible examples, a former Obama administration health official called Andy Slavitt predicted that just nine days from now, America's largest cities and hospitals would be 'overrun with cases,'" Tucker Carlson deadpanned into the camera during his prime-time Fox show on May 22, 2020.[1]

"Now, Slavitt is not an epidemiologist. In fact, he is a former McKinsey consultant. But countless other self-described 'experts' on television backed him up. A huge number of Americans, they told us, would get infected with the coronavirus, and a huge number would die, and die in the ugliest, most desperate way—gasping for breath with tubes shoved down their throats.

"Now, at the time, the World Health Organization suggested that a million Americans would die this way. The WHO estimated a case fatality rate of 3.4 percent. It's horrifying. It scared the hell out of the country. It scared the hell out of us. I think we repeated those numbers to you on this show."

Carlson continued: "But they were totally wrong. We now know, thanks to widespread blood testing, that the virus isn't that deadly. An enormous percentage of coronavirus infections produce mild symptoms or no symptoms at all. They're asymptomatic. The death toll is a tiny fraction of what we were told it would be."

At the time Carlson made those comments, more than 92,000 Americans had already died, but the rate of growth in the number of COVID-19 cases had taken a temporary dip. It would soon resurge, with new cases doubling over the next 45 days after Carlson's show.[2] As happened during these temporary dips, people like Carlson would emerge and label the entire pandemic a giant exaggeration and all but over. Even during these dips, hundreds more Americans were dying every day.

On his May 22 show, Carlson had gone on to mention New York governor Andrew Cuomo and Dr. Anthony Fauci as other alarmists who, along with me, had unnecessarily scared the American people. "At the time, ambitious politicians understood instinctively that Americans were really scared, and some did their best to heighten that fear," Carlson said. In other words, he was saying that Cuomo, Fauci, and I had done this purposely. As of that day, however, New York's death toll was 23,100.[3]

Carlson did offer some praise. It was for Kristi Noem, the governor of South Dakota, for having the backbone to refuse to close any businesses or issue a stay-at-home directive to quell the virus. Before long, South Dakota would become one of the world's biggest hot spots. With its relatively small population, under 900,000, South Dakota blew past South Korea with its population of over 50 million people in the number of deaths. By mid-November, almost 60 percent of tests for COVID-19 in South Dakota were coming back positive.[4]

If Americans were pandemic novices who didn't trust experts, that also made us clay to be molded by news personalities such as Carlson, as well as by those on social media and elsewhere who had other agendas. People like Carlson didn't provide the news as much as provide a reason to be angry about it or dismissive of it. To Carlson and those like him, the coronavirus was little more than a word, a concept; it was invisible, and therefore easy to distort.

Tucker's World vs. the Real World

Few people had a closer view of what COVID-19 actually looked like than Cleavon Gilman, an emergency medicine physician at New York–Presbyterian Hospital. The worst days in the emergency room during the pandemic seemed all too familiar to him. At age 19, after losing his father to an overdose, he had joined the navy as a hospital corpsman and eventually deployed to Iraq. He became a combat medic in a field hospital, stabilizing battlefield casualties before they were flown out for more treatment. After his tour, he found himself experiencing PTSD symptoms, such as fear and recurring memories of friends who had died in front of him. With the support of his family, he spent a decade rebuilding his resilience, though he couldn't have known just how much he would need it again.

When he left the navy, he promised himself he would never again put himself in a situation where he had to fear for his life. He became a physician so he could continue to help people, and found himself attracted to emergency medicine.

Then came February 2020. Medical professionals, like the rest of us, had for weeks been following reports of the outbreak of a new disease in Wuhan, China. One day, one of his fellow residents at New York–Presbyterian flagged him down in the hallway and said, "The virus is in Italy."

"Oh, it's in Italy?" Gilman responded. "Then it's already here." *People can't imagine that bad things will ever happen here,* he thought.

When the crush came to New York, it came fast. It was worse than Iraq. His hospital was intubating 20 patients a day. He was losing three a day. When, at long last, things in New York began to take a turn for the better, his colleagues finally took long-overdue breaks. He hoped they would have an opportunity to collect themselves so they didn't experience PTSD the way he had. Gilman thought about taking some time off himself.

But just as COVID-19 began lessening in the Northeast, it started springing up in other parts of the country. As tired and scarred as he was, Gilman realized he was still needed on the front lines, so when he heard about a job opening in an ER in Arizona, he signed on. He knew Arizona had no mask mandate, its bars and restaurants were open, and people spent too much time together indoors avoiding the heat. Because they hadn't seen a wave of virus the way the Northeast had, he knew, most Arizonans couldn't imagine it impacting them. But Gilman also knew that they were about to see their hometowns become battlefields. So he packed a bag and boarded a plane for Phoenix. From Phoenix, he headed for the border town of Yuma and his next mission, at Yuma Regional Medical Center. Months later, he was battling full ICUs. "You would think that the country would have learned its lesson, but I feel like 20,000 people that died in New York died for nothing."[5]

He blamed the propaganda fed to people from a safe distance from the front lines for distorting reality. He continued to read tweets from people saying COVID-19 was a giant exaggeration designed to scare people or make political points. It only reminded him how much people wanted to tune out unpleasantness and believe it would never affect them. He saw people attempt to spin the facts of situations they wouldn't get near in a million years leading to his full emergency rooms. But while Tucker Carlson continued his attack on the severity of the virus, Gilman began communicating in his own way. He began writing and posting simple profiles of people who had died from COVID-19. He wanted people to see the faces.

"The Reverse Goldilocks Virus"

The psychology of public reaction to the virus troubled me. It wasn't simply that many people distrusted experts. It was how many could justify not even doing small, simple things that would protect themselves and others. Bill Joy had said back in March that there were very low-tech ways to prevent this virus from spreading. The formula was within our grasp if we wanted it. All we had to do was not breathe on one another or congregate indoors. But many people felt that they were safe. They couldn't see the path the virus would be taking: big city to bedroom community to rural town, big venue to local tavern to family party. They didn't understand that fertile ground for the virus was any place where people didn't protect themselves from it. Perhaps worst of all, they discounted their role as a link in a chain that eventually passed the virus on to someone it did real damage to.

Some of this was easy to understand. The virus wasn't as constant a presence as the everyday things they missed from pre-pandemic days, like going to school, their business, or church, or socializing. Ed Yong referred to COVID-19 as "the reverse Goldilocks virus": just deadly enough to kill lots of people, but not so deadly as to force people to change their lifestyle or consider making a sustained sacrifice.

In hurricane season, governors often hold news conferences outdoors, rain slickers on, urging citizens to stay indoors to protect themselves and their property, or to get on the road and beat it out of town. But with a pandemic there is no threatening sky, no gusts of wind, no floodwaters. And afterward, as Ed pointed out, there are no submerged cars or downed trees to show that the storm has passed through. With a virus, we can't see the enemy or the damage—and our minds (and TV news channels) can mislead us into thinking there isn't any. Trading off even a small part of our lives for something we can't see requires a willful act of imagination and empathy.

When the global pandemic was still relatively new, the country did have a "we're all in this together" moment—cheering on our health care workforce in March and April, bringing out sewing machines to make masks, and marking the first few hundred deaths as they were announced on the news. These were as close to common experiences as the country experienced anymore. But little by little, Americans' patience waned. Trump and several Republican governors believed that they could focus on the economy without addressing public health, so many people let their guard down and assumed the worst was past. Subsequent bad news gave lots of people the feeling that this was more of a marathon than they had signed up for—particularly because they felt safe individually.

And individual circumstances affected how they viewed the pandemic: someone in a hard-hit area with an at-risk person in their household viewed it differently than did someone in another part of the country who had a small business at risk. There was no voice reminding people of their role in keeping the virus alive while it continued to do real damage.

If the president had stopped at "just" avoiding good public health guidelines, it would have been enough of a challenge. By fall, people all around the world were complaining of fatigue at complying with public health guidelines. But Trump took matters a step further and turned the decision about whether to wear a mask from a question of public health into a statement about freedom and liberty and what kind of American you were. National health care leaders in other countries told me this was one problem they were grateful not to have.

How Not to Have a Conversation About a Pandemic

By summer, the tone of the public conversation about the pandemic wasn't just confused or angry; it was getting downright scary. Simply for having a nuanced discussion of the pros and cons of mask wearing, prominent epidemiologist Mike Osterholm was getting threats from people who didn't like what he had to say. Some vowed to get his research defunded; others made physical threats serious enough that he turned them over to law enforcement.

Threats of physical violence to those who dared to contradict the president would soon become all too common. David Agus, a physician and scientist of very high regard who was working to help speed the development of safe vaccines, received a death threat from someone strongly opposed to vaccine use. Public health officials around the country began receiving death threats too, and many resigned. Many who didn't were shaken. And if you were the subject of a derisive tweet from the president, it became even more concerning. By the summer, Dr. Anthony Fauci couldn't go for his daily power walk without a federal security detail.[6]

Trump's influence over his followers became clear in other ways as well. At the end of March, the *New York Times* published a survey showing that Democrats were almost twice as concerned as Republicans about the coronavirus. Would there have been the same partisan difference under President George W. Bush, a president who recognized the threat of pandemics and who trusted experts? We'll never know. But there's no inherent reason for such a difference. To me, this reinforced the need to counteract Trump not with a Democratic message but with a nonpartisan one.[7]

I had spent months trying to take an approach without apportioning blame, both in private and in public. My private relationship with the Trump administration remained fairly constant. I kept trying to influence the course of how they managed the disease (though my success rate on that wasn't exactly world class), and I continued to answer any call for help they needed.

But with each passing week it became clearer to me that Trump had little interest in saving American lives, including those of his followers. In May he abandoned the states, sidelined the task force, and maligned public health measures. In June, with nearly 120,000 deaths already having occurred, he said, "The numbers are starting to get very good."[8] I found it more difficult to go on TV and not be critical of the president. Still, for most of the summer, even as I pointed out mistakes and held him accountable, I kept looking forward to that next life that could be saved.

Two things caused me to change course. The first was the release of the Bob Woodward interview tapes, which showed that Trump knew in January exactly how deadly the virus would be and still did nothing. He didn't just miscalculate or fail to understand. He went to bed every night knowing he was likely presiding over hundreds of thousands of preventable deaths.

The second was the coming election. Not all our problems would be solved by a new person in the Oval Office, but so many of them wouldn't be solved *without* a new person in the Oval Office. I only assisted the Biden campaign and the transition team in the most tangential of ways—whenever I was asked to, or when there were things they needed to be ready for—but I knew most of the health care team who would be assisting Biden if he won, and in my view, the sooner we had a change, the better for the country.

I still believed that public health was not a partisan issue. As I saw Trump work against the public interest, I made a point of increasing media appearances with other Republicans like Scott Gottlieb and Mark McClellan. I never stopped working with people in the Trump White House if I thought it would help, but when it came to public restraint, finally I'd had enough. On September 9, in response to the Woodward revelation, I tweeted, "I don't like COVID threads about Donald Trump. But sometimes there is no choice. Today there is no choice. . . . Trump's defenders like to say, 'It wouldn't have been any different under Obama.' It would have been different under anyone but a madman."[9]

Atlas Shrugged It Off

There's only so many ways to say "it's ok for some people to die" without sounding like an asshole.
—Andy Slavitt on Twitter, May 8, 2020[10]

Dr. Scott Jensen, a Republican state senator from Minnesota, was a primary care doctor who had developed several interesting theories. At the end of March, he posted a video to Facebook to reassure us that while 40,000 Americans die of the flu every year, only 800 had died from the coronavirus. He held up a golf ball and an M&M and said the flu was like the golf ball and COVID-19 was like the M&M. The media eagerly sought out "contrarians" like Jensen, who in turn was eager for national attention. Soon he turned up on Laura Ingraham's Fox News show floating the idea that because doctors and hospitals received a higher Medicare payment for patients with COVID-19 diagnoses, they might be falsifying their numbers of coronavirus cases and deaths.[11]

I had worked with Jensen on a couple of health care issues in the Minnesota state legislature. I had indeed found him to be a contrarian and someone who liked the sound of his own voice a little too much. He'd come over to my house one day for a conversation and to deliver a self-published book on health care he thought I should read.

One day in late March 2020, after seeing a livestreamed town hall he did—indoors, while sitting maskless and within a few feet of another Republican state senator, and where he minimized the threat of COVID-19—I called him.[12] He had just ended the town hall. I questioned whether this was the example he wanted to be setting. He responded that he was a physician and believed COVID-19 was just like a flu.

I asked him what data he had seen. He hadn't seen any, but instead inquired about data I had seen.

There was plenty of data to indicate how different COVID-19 was from the flu, from infectiousness to hospitalizations to the death rate. But I didn't mention it.

I just said, "Scott, why don't we both simply ask people to follow Jan's advice so we don't confuse them? Let's not create all these alternate authorities. Let's count on her to interpret the data and make recommendations." Jan Malcolm was the Minnesota state health commissioner. "We don't understand this thing yet." But Malcolm was a Democrat, and Jensen told me he wasn't about to defer to her.

I pointed him to other Republicans who were saying responsible things about the threat of the virus. He told me we had a "difference in views."

There was indeed a difference. "Your views are dangerous, Scott."

To some people, Scott Jensen and Scott Atlas looked like authorities. They are physicians, after all. Never mind that they have only a little more experience with virology or epidemiology than any of the rest of us. In fact, in a broad and unevenly traveling pandemic, they brought a myopic view fixed on a belief in their own experience—which was far more dangerous than having no data at all but an open mind. The WHO coined the term "infodemic" to describe the rapid and far-reaching spread of false information in regard to the coronavirus.[13]

More than anything, the lack of humility and the confidence of the people who wanted to downplay the pandemic were impressive.

The BSer-in-chief was, of course, Trump himself. A study by researchers at Cornell University analyzed 38 million news articles about the pandemic and found that 38 percent of misinformation about the virus was generated by no one other than Trump. As if undermining the CDC weren't enough, Trump commonly retweeted conspiracy theorists who called COVID-19 a "plandemic" (a term coined by filmmaker Mikki Willis, who produced a controversial documentary on COVID-19), began rumors about Dr. Anthony Fauci purposely injecting poison, and suggested that only a few thousand people had actually died from COVID-19.[14]

The most dangerous kinds of deniers were those who actively pushed a theory that we should allow the infection to spread so that society could reach herd immunity. Herd immunity (or "herd mentality," as Trump once ironically referred to it) happens when a large enough percentage of the population becomes immune to a disease, which in turn diminishes the spread of the disease.[15] The Mayo Clinic estimated that 70 percent of Americans would need to be either infected with COVID-19 or vaccinated in order to achieve herd immunity.[16]

There is perhaps no greater contrast to Hubert H. Humphrey's challenge to govern morally than those who called for herd immunity. White House advisor Scott Atlas and the Koch-funded American Institute for Economic Research (AIER) were the loudest voices advocating for this approach. In a document known as the Great Barrington Declaration, the AIER summed it up bluntly: "Those who are not vulnerable should immediately be allowed to resume life as normal." They called for no actual safety measures other than to "protect older people." Like many populist calls, it had its enticing elements—it required no effort, and it allowed people to go about their everyday lives with a clear conscience. But, in fact, this approach was supported by people whose main interest was individual liberty unfettered by the government.[17]

Referring to the Great Barrington Declaration in October, Atlas's support was unqualified. "We're not endorsing the plan. The plan is endorsing what the president's policy has been for months," he said.[18]

People who promote herd immunity often make a point of saying the elderly should be protected, which of course gives the theory an air of reasonableness. But herd immunity is a surefire path to illness and death, *particularly* among the most vulnerable populations. It is impossible to separate the low-risk and high-risk populations. As noted earlier, only 6.5 percent of the elderly live separately from the general population in congregate care settings, and most people with health conditions that put them at increased risk (heart disease, type 2 diabetes, obesity, cancer, autoimmune diseases, and so on) also don't live separately. A full 40 percent of the public was at high risk.[19] Sweden, the country whose approach most closely resembles a herd immunity strategy, found it impossible to protect its elderly population.

Looking at the idea for even 15 minutes revealed that the notion of herd immunity defied any sense of morality or logic. When Atlas made his statement about the Great Barrington Declaration, only 10 percent of the population had been infected (and presumably had some immunity) and over 200,000 people had died.[20] If you believe the Mayo Clinic's estimate, herd immunity (in the absence of a vaccine) would require hundreds of thousands more Americans to needlessly die. And while Charles Koch has a spacious place to live safe from infection, the herd immunity proposal over-looked how many people like Ahmed Aden there were, forced to live in tight quarters with people who were especially vulnerable to the virus. Sure enough, by November, nursing home deaths alone crossed 100,000 across the United States.[21] There is another, more accurate name for herd immunity that its proponents didn't dare use: herd thinning.

Promoting herd immunity wasn't just ineffective and cruel; it was also, frankly, risky and stupid. Because no one understood how long immunity to COVID-19 lasted, it was entirely possible that 25 percent of the population would become infected early on, only to find a year later that they were no longer immune. Even in 2020, before the emergence of mutant strains that resisted antibodies from prior infections, there were several well-documented cases in which one bout of COVID-19 was followed in the same individual by a second bout of a different strain.[22] And, of course, the long-term effects of being exposed to the virus were not well understood. What was known is that the virus was capable of causing structural damage to virtually any organ, the clotting system, the immune system, or the limbs. And while the virus would remain incompletely understood for a long time, there was a much simpler path for dealing with it, as this book outlines: follow what had been done successfully in the rest of the world.

Masks, Trump Rallies, and Stoking the Culture Wars

In April, while masks were still not being promoted to the public, and vaccines were a long way off, I wrote that we already had the best preventative technology right in front of our noses:[23]

> If there is a silver bullet, it may not be a vaccine or therapy that outsmarts the virus. There's a scenario where the virus is destroyed completely by something far simpler—a reusable, cleanable, highly functional, and nearly free mask. Viruses can't survive with no-

where to go. Cutting the virus off at the pass may be most simply done by never letting the droplets get into the air. . . . Even if you don't welcome the idea of wearing a mask for a period of time (and I would argue, why not?), the larger point is we are not powerless in the face of this virus. We have science, ingenuity, and collective action.

When we breathe or speak, we generate respiratory droplets that are between 50 and 100 micrometers in size. Any of those droplets, should they contain a sufficient viral load of the coronavirus, can lodge in someone's lungs, and from there the virus can travel throughout the body, causing all manner of damage. But face coverings get in the way. A comprehensive review of the research found that depending on the fabric and construction, cloth masks filter out between 49 percent and 86 percent of small particles. Surgical masks filter out 89 percent, and N95 masks filter out 95 percent. A cloth mask has been demonstrated to be highly effective at protecting other people in the vicinity of the mask wearer, while surgical and N95 masks protect the wearer and others.[24]

Before it was well understood that asymptomatic people could spread the virus, major scientific institutions supported limiting mask wearing to health care workers and people with symptoms. Once we discovered more about how the virus was transmitted, masks became more available, and the initial mask mandates were put in place across the United States, growth rates slowed by an average of 1 percent daily. In a study comparing mask-wearing practices across 198 countries, the mortality rate from COVID-19 in those countries where mask wearing was either government policy or cultural norm increased by 8 percent per week on average, compared to 54 percent per week for countries that did not encourage mask wearing. A report by the IHME released in late October 2020 estimated that 130,000 lives could be saved in the United States between fall of that year and spring 2021 if people universally wore masks. This was a constant truth of the pandemic: saving lives was always possible if we chose to do it.[25]

In the United States, the clearer it became that protective masks would save lives, the harder people in some quarters resisted wearing them. Trump had a large role to play in this both because of what he did and because of what he did not do. He mocked reporters who wore masks and he did not require staffers or attendees at his rallies or indoor events to wear masks. Several of those events became hot spots or superspreader events, most famously Trump's nomination ceremony for Supreme Court justice Amy Coney Barrett in late September.

On October 11, my first call of the day was from Mike DeWine, the Republican governor of Ohio. Cases across Ohio were growing at a very high rate, almost entirely in rural parts of the state. DeWine had put a mask mandate in place. He estimated there was 90 percent mask use compliance in the cities, but it was far lower in the rural areas.

He wasn't calling to ask whether a mask mandate was the right thing. The science was clear on that. Trump officials including Brett Giroir, Anthony Fauci, Deborah Birx, surgeon general Jerome Adams, and a host of other scientists agreed. A month earlier, CDC chair Robert Redfield had testified in a Senate hearing that "this face mask is more guaranteed to protect me against COVID than when I take a COVID vaccine." Rather, DeWine was calling because, as a Republican, he took a lot of heat for his mask mandate, which Fox News denigrated as an attack on freedom, and he wanted to discuss ideas on how to address blowback from the public against mask wearing. DeWine believed his first duty was the safety of the people in his state. We ended up talking for a half hour almost entirely about communication, sociology, and public engagement.[26]

As I had written a few days earlier in the *Journal of the American Medical Association*, "In the US, people are comfortable with and accustomed to scientists rescuing them or helping them avoid disaster. But when that does not work perfectly, or leaves temporary gaps, people are left to rely on something less predictable—the human psyche and human interaction—to prevent the spread of the virus."[27]

"How do I convince people in rural areas to wear masks?" DeWine asked.

"I think we have to be creative and hear people out," I advised him. "People don't like to be told what to do."

"But I need to keep the mask mandate. We can show it's increased mask wearing and is working in urban locations. I'm afraid making compliance voluntary would be interpreted as saying it's okay not to wear a mask."

"I wouldn't suggest that, but, even with a mandate, you still have a sales job. You might want to create ways to engage people in safe activities—smaller gatherings, forums for people to do something rather than being told what to do, get local organizations involved. If we think this is going to go beyond a few months, we need a sustainable strategy."

Seven months into the pandemic, the good news was that the public health science was settled. But DeWine and other politicians were now encountering new obstacles: the country's frustration and fatigue, the politics, and a culture war.

While Trump's supporters actively flouted mask use compliance, and Republican politicians such as North Carolina gubernatorial candidate Dan Forest ran on a platform of "no mask mandate," Trump's approach was more playful—and more careful. If pressed, he would say that people were welcome to wear masks if they wanted to, but he'd add a giant wink. On the evening of my call with Mike DeWine, Trump held a political rally in Washington where he both tossed masks to the crowd and said, "I'll kiss everyone." At the Capitol that day, his chief of staff, Mark Meadows, made a show of dramatically stepping far back from reporters and taking off his mask before smirking and walking away. These cues weren't lost on the public.[28] Of course, neither Trump nor Meadows avoided getting sick and spreading COVID-19 themselves.

Clusterf*** at the White House

On October 1, 2020, the world learned that Donald Trump had tested positive for COVID-19. Everything that happened from then on was a microcosm of virtually everything the president had done to date to deny and avoid dealing with the virus. First he appeared to blame his infection on a staffer, Hope Hicks. When that was no longer tenable, he blamed it on Gold Star families he had met with. Then he denied that his illness amounted to much. Soon after he was admitted to Walter Reed Medical Center, the White House physician, Sean Conley, misled the public about the severity of the president's illness—describing it as mild, even as it worsened and doctors were pumping Trump with drug cocktails not yet available to the general public as well as a number of other powerful medications.[29]

The circumstances surrounding how Trump had acquired the virus and whom he spread it to were also kept purposely murky. The White House would not confirm the timing of when Trump first knew he had caught the virus. What was clear was that Trump participated in a number of indoor events without a mask before, during, and after the time when he knew Hicks had tested positive and he had been exposed to her. He knowingly endangered staffers as well as donors he met with during a fundraiser at his Bedminster, New Jersey, golf club, and possibly donors at events in Minnesota as well. During his stay at Walter Reed Medical Center, Trump insisted on a jaunt in a hermetically sealed car with several Secret Service personnel enclosed in the space with him.[30] The Secret Service later had a significant outbreak.[31]

There are even more troubling elements to Trump's reaction to the illness and his lack of concern for the safety of others. The same goes for the White House staff. Within a few weeks of Trump's diagnosis, the infections of at least 40 people—staffers, guests, aides, and reporters—could be traced to the White House.[32] Still, the White House did not contact people who'd been exposed to the president or to other staffers who tested positive. The White House turned down an offer from the CDC to conduct a full contact tracing regime.

Michael Shear has been a White House correspondent for the *New York Times* since 2008. The White House has been his place of work longer than it has been Donald Trump's. On October 1, Michael fell ill with symptoms he knew to be COVID-19. He had never been contacted by the White House to let him know he had been exposed. As he was recovering, I asked him what this said about the president; he demurred. I then reminded him that the White House was his office as much as it was the president's. Finally Shear said, "The core difference is that I can't imagine other presidents being so disdainful of the scientific advice that they were getting. That then led to this really incredible divide between the scientific community and the ruling leadership."[33]

The White House created a cloud around questions that any one of us would be expected to answer: Who was exposed to whom when? When were they tested and when did they know? How many people did staffers infect? How many people did the president infect?

Trump's medical care also revealed a great deal about the unequal health care system in the United States. Trump had access to what he later called a "miracle cure," which was actually a cocktail of monoclonal antibodies, a promising but very expensive therapy, which at the time was not available to other patients even through an emergency use authorization.

The president's carelessness with the lives of those around him was on full display through every step of his illness. In April 2020, after British prime minister Boris Johnson contracted COVID-19 and spent time in the intensive care unit, he called the virus "an unexpected and invisible mugger" and became insistent about a national virus-control policy. Trump, on the other hand, told Americans, "Don't be afraid of COVID. I'm immune, I feel great."[34]

Closing the Compassion Gap

This book documents how we mishandled the pandemic and let many things get in the way of controlling the spread of the virus. But everyone who puts forward an opinion got plenty wrong along the way. That certainly includes me. Because of that, humility was essential—but it was often missing.

I didn't try to hold myself up as an expert, but rather tried to amplify the voices of those people who knew the most. But occasionally I veered into thinking I knew more than I did. Approximately once each month, I would try to document publicly on Twitter the things I had been wrong about. If I had to pick what I was most wrong about, it wouldn't be what I have sometimes been called out for: when I tweeted that according to experts a million people could die from this. Sadly, those experts were justified. Rather, what I got most wrong was how people would respond to the unprecedented mass deaths of their fellow Americans. I had believed we would unite in our grief. I had thought the pandemic could bring us together. But our attention was fleeting, we got numbed by statistics, and the country met death tolls we had never seen before with an almost casual indifference. Ed Yong described it as "a catastrophic lack of empathy." And I agree. As he said, many Americans felt *just* safe enough from the virus, and *just* burdened enough by the privations.

It isn't just hundreds of thousands of us who have died. It's that each death represents years of life taken away. A researcher at Harvard estimated in October that up to that point, the coronavirus had deprived people of 2.5 million years of potential life in the United States alone—"years that might otherwise have been filled with . . . trips to the grocery store, late night conversations on the phone, tearful firsts with a newborn baby." Many of those years of life could have been saved.[35]

One day in mid-September, I called Andy Beshear, the Democratic first-term governor of Kentucky; at one point he enjoyed an 82 percent favorability rating for his handling of the coronavirus, one of the highest in the nation. His father, Steve Beshear, was a former governor, and also had been one of the most successful health care governors in the country. During the elder Beshear's administration, the uninsured rate in Kentucky declined from 20 percent to 8 percent, improving hundreds of thousands of lives.[36] Andy Beshear was a newer model of his father: bright, open-minded, a listener, accountable, and decent.

Andy's approach had been to try something unusual and old-fashioned: call on people to sacrifice for one another. "'The greatest generation' is already taken," he told me. "We will get through this by being 'the kindest generation.'"[37]

He went on: "For us, it's a different set of skills. Do we have what it takes to continue doing the right things? . . . Are we willing to make personal sacrifices to save the lives of those around us? We've seen some really callous examples of suggesting just because people are older, that the loss of life isn't tragic, and the loss of eight to ten years with a family isn't important. It is."

Kentucky, a poor state, had managed to achieve one of the lowest death rates in the country. Even so, several businesses filed a lawsuit against the mask mandate he'd implemented. There were people carrying signs in the capital saying Beshear was "drunk with power."

If I'm ever drunk with power, I plan to choose something more imaginative than making people wear a mask.

My dad used to say that America was a place where you could see both the most beautiful and the ugliest. The quiet charity and the loud violence and hate. The bravery and the bullying. That's never more true than in our moments of great crisis.

I've discussed one reason why I think other countries do better in responding to pandemics—previous experience with infectious diseases. It far outweighs travel restrictions or proximity to the pandemic's origins. Hong Kong, for example, has more cross-border travel to and from Wuhan, where the virus originated, than anyplace else, but as of October 2020 only 105 people there had died. That's very likely because Hong Kong, like Japan, Singapore, and the Democratic Republic of Congo, had faced epidemics before (in Hong Kong's case, a flu epidemic in 1968 and the SARS epidemic in 2003).

But there's another reason other countries have done better than we have, and it isn't wealth and resources. As of November, why did the United States, the wealthiest country in the world, suffer 70 deaths per 100,000 people, while Haiti, ranked 145th in wealth, had only 2 deaths per 100,000? Wealth itself was generally a much worse predictor of a country's pandemic resilience than wealth equality. Australia, Norway, Finland, and Denmark, all more egalitarian countries than the United States, all have had death rates around 10 or below per 100,000. On the other hand, countries with extremes of both wealth and poverty have had much higher death rates, with Saudi Arabia and Russia at the low end of that group with 15 and 20 deaths per 100,000 population, respectively, and Brazil near the United States at the top, with 77.[38] And places with strong social ties, like Japan, Singapore, Hong Kong, and New Zealand, had rates far, far lower.

Andy Beshear believed that, rather than fighting the other side, the better path was to ask for sacrifice.

> I do think that we've learned here that when you really need people to do something, but that something is sometimes to do nothing, it is more emotionally challenging than if we'd ask people to head into the factories like we like we did during World War II. What we're asking of people really here is so little compared to what we've had to in the past. But emotionally and in terms of anxiety, it may be even more difficult. This virus is mean and how it attacks our human psyche and our emotions. But we're strong and we just have to be committed.[39]

Being called upon for something greater, being asked to do something to contribute—was this not how we in the United States thought of ourselves? Was it not who we aspired to be? In past times of great crisis, didn't people come together? Put aside differences? Or was that vision long gone? Had that vision been possible only in a type of society that no longer existed here in the United States—a more intimate society, a more homogenous society?

Beyond the obvious failure of leadership, what was different this time?

CHAPTER 12

THE WORK TO DO

SCENE: PLANET EARTH

It was a 28-degree October Saturday, 10 days before the presidential election. I showered and eschewed my work-at-home uniform of sweatpants and a hoodie for clothes with zippers and buttons. Brodie followed me downstairs, but when, for the first time in six months, I bypassed my office and headed for the garage and the barely familiar feel of my car, he shot me a look of betrayal.

My 90-minute drive to Rochester, Minnesota, that day was sparked by a request from Deborah Birx. Birx had failed to persuade the president to address the virus, and with Scott Atlas's arrival she had been cast out of the inner circle entirely. Now she was back working with her old boss, Anthony Fauci, and the people in the CDC to limit what she saw as the ongoing horror. Her colleagues there were producing reports showing that the spread of the virus was picking up steam heading into the fall and winter and that it was reaching communities that were unprepared for its arrival. She was at this point touring the country, visiting state after state and issuing dire warnings. Her regular routine was to fly into airports with a staff member or two and drive around the local area—to colleges, shops, farmers' markets, and anywhere she could observe people—and finish with a meeting with local officials. She'd also begun sending out her weekly report, "The Governor's Report," which, according to Ryan P., included the best and most detailed information that existed about the indicators of spread.

She had arranged a small meeting with school superintendents in Minnesota and had reached out to Governor Walz's team. She'd also asked that Mike Osterholm and I meet her there and sit in on the meeting.

These meetings reminded me of the many road shows I had done during my time in government: U-shaped tables, a tight invitation list of local officials and advocates, people showing up with messages ready to deliver. Birx's MO at these events was to hold an hour-long meeting and then do a readout for the local press to share what the data was telling her and hope to drive some action.

Upon my arrival at Rochester Community and Technical College, I was ushered into what had become a classic post-COVID meeting setup: extra-large rooms, chairs spaced, hand sanitizer by each name card, everyone wearing masks the entire time, no handshakes. There was no Saturday version of Birx in jeans and a sweatshirt; she was dressed smartly, with her signature scarf, and displayed few visible signs of weariness. But she was blunt.

"Fighting the virus and Scott Atlas together is the hardest thing I've had to do," she said.

She was speaking for all of us at this point. Only in place of "Scott Atlas," she could have substituted any number of names or phrases—he was an avatar for so many things. She could have said "fatigue" or "anti-science" or "inequality." A lot of Americans could have said "a country that doesn't have my back" or "fear of the future." It's never been about just the virus.

We haven't lightened people's loads during the pandemic. We have piled on.

I had watched Deborah Birx over the months and occasionally been in touch with her. I'd seen her cycle through different phases: at some points sunny and hopeful, at others compliant and silent, sometimes creative and strategic, and occasionally pounding the table and barely able to hide her disgust. At the end of October 2020, she was beyond all of that; she was downright scared. In the period between mid-March and the end of April, her bosses had been paying modest attention. During that time, she played the game to fit in more in the White House culture. But like every one of Trump's handpicked leaders with scientific credentials—including FDA commissioner Stephen Hahn, CDC director Robert Redfield, surgeon general Jerome Adams, and Anthony Fauci—as Trump became more overt in his self-serving neglect and manipulation, her mild protests left her out in the cold. She began to quietly hammer away at whatever she could affect. Well-meaning but overwhelmed by the politics of the White House, she now seemed on a desperate effort for redemption.

By this time, though, Birx was no longer allowed at the podium at White House press conferences. These trips she was making were the only sanctioned national effort left. Now we were battling a disease that spread in all directions at blinding and invisible speed with analog printouts and a team traveling to one town at a time. As the virus raced, our only national response was forced to move glacially and in relative secret.

With cases ramping up around the country and hospitals beginning to fill again, her message that day was different from the administration's. "We are out of time," she said. "I can't just say that, but we have no time."

"You can say it," Osterholm objected, not a creature of anyone's politics. "People just want the truth. They want to know how they protect themselves."

We were indeed about to be in for an onslaught of deaths that dwarfed anything we had seen before. The death toll would double over the next three months. Yet, there was no press conference, no public warning, and no action from the president or his staff.[1]

At the end of the meeting with the school superintendents, as others filed out, I stood to talk to Birx, masked and six feet distant.

I wanted to get a sense for whether, in the event of a strained transition of government, she would help give Biden and his team the best chance to be effective.

At one point, after a brief pause, she looked me in the eye and said, "I hope the election turns out a certain way." I had the most important information I needed.

Later that day she texted me a thank-you. I invited her on my podcast to talk with me about the upcoming Thanksgiving holiday, which we were both concerned about and which she had referred to as potential 35 million superspreader events.

She responded, "I am completely silenced. They let me do these local trips and local media, but no national media. Makes me crazy. But I summarize the data every morning, and it goes up the chain and to Tony [Fauci], so he has everything." Other than a brief chat when Trump was ill, it had been months since Fauci had spoken to the president. Unlike Birx, he kept enough of his voice and did join me on the podcast.

It was one thing for me to feel like all I could do was to keep focusing on saving the next life. It was another thing for the highest-ranking scientist on the White House's own task force to feel entirely defeated. I wondered if Birx felt she had failed. She had spent the last year inside someone else's make-believe world. Things had turned out far, far worse than she had anticipated back in March, when she'd believed the IHME's projection of a total of 60,000 deaths in the United States. In public service, like in many things, you can spend a lot of time rationalizing things when they don't go well and blaming all the constraints. Occasionally you have moments when you think about what you could have done differently. I wondered what she regretted.

"I have no illusions about my career in government," she had confided in me. She had to know her reputation had been damaged by some of her mistakes and compromises she no doubt felt she'd needed to make. Her pilgrimage on the road these last few months seemed almost a religious effort at redemption, a long slow journey to attempt to do justice to the truths that had been destroyed so thoroughly over the year.

Chimera

In the late 1980s, the Soviets had launched "Hunter," a secret biowarfare program to develop what is known as a chimera.[2] A chimera is an organism containing DNA from multiple other organisms. The project's aim was to combine DNA from equine encephalitis, smallpox, and Ebola into a potent biological weapon capable of killing 100 million people if released in the United States. The Soviet biological weapons program had begun in the 1920s and was infamous for its size, its sophistication, and its secrecy. But Hunter was unique in that it aimed to combine the worst properties of lethality (Ebola) and infectiousness (smallpox) into one. Imagining a bug like this focuses the mind—think of something that spreads with great speed and kills most of the people who come in contact with it.

COVID-19 is not a Hunter-level chimera by a long shot. If it were, our lack of preparation would have been far more costly. But what if our next pandemic is? What if it attacks in a way that is even more lethal than COVID-19, or more contagious, or both? What if it doesn't prey on the elderly but, like the measles, preys on children?

This is not just idle speculation. Blythe Adamson's bedtime story isn't a fairy tale. As our climate changes, and as we increasingly encroach on the habitats of other species, more odd things will happen. More viruses that we've never seen before will emerge.

When the next pandemic comes, will we hold out for a silver bullet, or will we make pragmatic sacrifices? Will the next generation of Nancy Messonniers, Peter Markses, Rick Brights, and Anthony Faucis still be attracted to a career as civil servants? Will we ignore experts and turn against them, or will we let them inform and guide us? Will our definition of freedom include protecting the institutions that are at the heart of a free society? If we treat COVID-19 as our starter bug and take the right lessons from it, we stand a chance.

Reforms

What lessons should we take from all of our experiences with the pandemic beyond what we can say about the actions of one president?

When I sat down to write this last part of this book, I started with the belief that I owed readers a long list of reforms I wished to see: better ways of setting up government, investments in people and programs, safeguards, fixes to the health care system, reinvigoration of our scientific institutions, having Congress better support people displaced by the virus, and connecting to other countries around the world. I have published articles on these topics, as have many others, and that work and thinking will continue.

If you've read through the book, you know what some of these reforms are, and I've summarized them conveniently in an appendix, which I've labeled Exhibit N. The "N" stands for "Never," because the things listed in this exhibit will never happen—unless we do something to make them happen. Real, lasting reforms will require consensus. And they will require that we address parts of our society that have been problems for too long, including racial injustice, income inequality, and the negative consequences of capitalism itself. Let's face it: the pandemic showed us some of our ugly, and we should think about starting there.

As much as we may like to think so, the pandemic alone will not be enough to bring about these changes. Our system of government is designed to put brakes on change that happens too rapidly. And change that takes place too quickly or without consensus often begets a backlash. There are plenty of people—most of them very influential—who are comfortable with things just the way they are. We need what Ed Yong refers to as "radical introspection" if some of the deeper, more sweeping changes are to take hold. And we also need to do what Obama suggested to me when he called me in the middle of the fight to save the ACA: organize.

Am I certain that even if we did everything in Exhibit N we would avoid a bad outcome? I am not. I have no doubt we will have better leadership the next time we face a crisis like this. But if our first line of defense fails us, no set of policies will protect us if we don't make the underlying society work better. America isn't just an old house that needs a lengthy list of repairs. America is a conversation. To be healthy as a country, we need to figure out how to do something we are failing at more and more: talking to each other.

There are rights we hold dear, including the freedom not to be told by the government what to do. But throughout our history as a nation we have agreed to some restrictions in the name of a safer society. Sometimes we have competing values, but with enough experience, we can work through those so that society wins out. For example, seat belt laws were resisted but ultimately deemed important. It turned out that it wasn't a new law, but developing and spreading a culture of safety that was the more consequential result of the effort. Designated drivers, mandatory airbags and other standard safety features, and helmet laws all sprang from this culture of safety and have reduced unnecessary traffic deaths. But there had to be pioneers in that movement. Changes that ask each of us to sacrifice a little so that we can all gain a lot need a place to hatch.

As I initially finish writing this book toward the end of 2020, I have no inkling of what's to come, either for the country or for me (I reflect on those surprises in the Afterword). I can remind future readers of the feeling of still being very much in the middle of the worst of COVID-19 with only vague ideas about how it might resolve itself. Conditions are grim, the country tired, our health care workforce sorely abused, and broad availability of vaccines still months away. All the uncertainty is taking an extraordinary toll on many. But I know that eventually we will begin to recover from the trauma. There are many possible directions in which we can go as a nation, but it feels like they fall into two broad categories, and those lead us in two very different directions.

Death of a Society

In 2017, the TV producer Kayla Chadwick wrote a much-read opinion piece for the *Huffington Post* titled "I Don't Know How to Explain to You That You Should Care About Other People."[3] She writes, "If making sure your fellow citizens can afford to eat, get an education, and go to the doctor isn't enough of a reason to fund [a higher minimum wage, public education, and universal health care], I have nothing left to say to you." She made it clear how difficult it was to have effective policies if we cannot fundamentally agree on what we owe each other.

I would be surprised if we don't succeed at the most literal lessons from the pandemic. Being stocked up on PPE, for example, likely won't be a problem next time. The challenge will lie with the less literal lessons. We will have to do better than sigh in relief once this is behind us, with a blue-ribbon bipartisan commission putting out watered-down recommendations after a number of months behind closed doors.

The changes we need require a level of compassion and empathy that has been declining across our increasingly large, diverse, and fractured nation. There is not a lot to be confident about in that regard. We already tolerate plenty of preventable deaths. We have grown used to mass shootings in schools, churches, synagogues, nightclubs, and concerts. When a gunman killed 20 kindergartners and first graders at Sandy Hook Elementary School in 2012 and Congress refused to act in its wake, British journalist Dan Hodges tweeted that this "marked the end of the US gun control debate. Once America decided killing children was bearable, it was over." We have tolerated very uneven justice: Black Americans die at the hands of the police at 3.5 times the rate of whites. We have decided that it is acceptable for Americans to go without access to food or medicine: 40 million American kids go to bed hungry every night, and about one in four of us can't afford the prescriptions we need to stay healthy.[4]

A raging suicide and overdose epidemic was growing even before the pandemic. More than 67,000 people died of overdoses in 2018, and more than 48,000 people killed themselves, with very little in the way of public response.[5] Each time we experience these losses and do nothing to prevent the next ones, callousness becomes more baked in to our baseline and life in our free society takes a hit.

The same has held true in the pandemic. It was true after 10 people died, after 10,000 people died, and after 100,000 people died: had we had the will, on any given day we could have begun to dramatically reduce the virus's spread over the course of six to eight weeks—anytime we chose to care enough about the next life.

We don't need to solve all of society's ills to respond better to a pandemic, but we will have to do more than invest in a better first line of defense—we will need to break our pattern of indifference. Increasingly the American response to adversity can be defined by "Take care of your own. Everyone for themselves." If kids get shot, buy your own gun. If the climate changes, blame the people who live on low ground or near forests for not moving. The most tempting route post-pandemic will be to try to retreat back to normal as quickly as possible—for those who can. For some of those people, the biggest lessons they take away may be to stock up on more necessities, move into gated communities, and try to build better barriers to the intruding world through tougher immigration policies and more protectionism.

In 1842, Edgar Allan Poe wrote a short story called "The Masque of the Red Death."[6] Its protagonist, Prince Prospero, attempts to avoid a dangerous plague by retreating to a locked and fortified abbey with his wealthy and privileged friends. One night after five or six months in seclusion, he throws a masquerade ball for them. A guest appears dressed as the corpse of someone who has succumbed to the plague. The guest causes Prospero and the rest of his guests to get the plague, and they all soon die. Any story that ends with "And Darkness and Decay and the Red Death held illimitable dominion over all" is not a happy one . . . yikes.

This is what the death of a society looks like. When there's a pandemic, we blame scientists. When there are raging fires, we blame the forest. In a crisis, we try to protect ourselves and maybe even a neighbor or two, but for all the people we don't know personally, we suggest that a lack of "individual responsibility" is the culprit. If this crisis didn't harm us, we decide the next one won't harm us either, and so we never make the modest investment to prevent it. Instead, we chalk up massive losses to the cost of doing business. But every choice we make that ignores the suffering of others means we are that much less prepared for the next adversity when it arrives. And as Poe's tale relates, we are never completely safe or separate from the dangers our neighbors face. The most damaging blows to our society will be a series of retreats from collective responsibility. In the end, it won't take a chimera to knock us over; we will take care of that on our own.

A Society Renewed

There is, of course, another path, where the deeper lessons of the pandemic lead us to aim to fix what is broken. Society doesn't change by fiat or even by law. We change when attitudes change. Where does that process start? How would our civic leaders, faith leaders, and public champions begin that conversation? It would begin with mourning those we have lost. And it would mean inviting everyone to participate in that healing. Grieving those we've lost to COVID-19, of course, but also grieving the lost businesses and the lost school years and those we lost to suicide and overdoses. It would mean honoring those we have never fully thanked: doctors, EMTs, and nurses who held our loved ones' hands; laborers, farmworkers, drivers, and clerks who kept showing up; scientists and civil servants who occupied their posts and didn't quit on us and have that much more knowledge ready for the next time. Honoring them would start with listening to *them* telling us what has to be different next time.

If we wait for the next pandemic to make changes, we will be missing some important opportunities to address what has been shoved right in our faces: The kids who can't get enough to eat when they are away from school, or who can't study because they lack access to the internet at home. Those of us who live in crowded or unsafe places. Those of us living on the edge of a mental health crisis. Those of us who are isolated every day. Those of us who can't afford health care. We allowed people to live like this before the pandemic, and many more lived like this during the pandemic; it's up to us whether people live like this after the pandemic.

The Minnesota town that I live in has a tradition. When a family loses a school-age child, after the memorial service, as the family gets in their car and drives home from the burial, on every lamppost and every tree they pass is a balloon of their child's favorite color, thousands of them, for miles if need be, tied on during the service by people from all over town. The balloons lead all the way to their driveway, where dozens more balloons flank their home. On occasions when you happen to be driving back from the store and you see balloons out, it freezes your insides. It becomes impossible to finish your cell phone conversation, listen to the radio, or argue with your kids in the backseat. And after the family has gone into their home for the evening, the same moms and dads and children who put the balloons up come back to take them down one by one.

If a global pandemic and hundreds of thousands of lost souls all feel too big to comprehend, we can see the pandemic as just many neighborhood tragedies. The act of helping people through the difficult times is healing, and the act of asking for help and receiving it is a powerful and affirming experience. None of us has the power to fix the entire pandemic or save every life. I had that pointed out to me several times throughout this crisis in my moments of deepest frustration. But I have just as much hope and determination as I had before. If we focus on saving the next life, helping the next neighbor, I think we improve our chances at tackling a good chunk of Exhibit N.

Even then, we won't get everyone on board. Societies never do. We will need to learn to disagree without turning into enemies. We have to keep including everyone in the conversation. Excluding the people we disagree with is not supposed to be a privilege of being in the majority.

But calling for inclusiveness isn't the same thing as calling for false agreement. Evil and selfishness will always be around. And sometimes they will occupy positions of authority at the exact wrong time.

As Deborah Birx and I parted on that Saturday in Rochester, I addressed a question she asked about what to do about Scott Atlas. I said, "There's no choice. We will just need to win." And I walked to my car and drove home.

AFTERWORD

WHAT HAPPENED NEXT

SCENE: WHITE HOUSE, MARCH 2021

On Saturday, November 7, after a highly contested election in which tens of millions of Americans voted by mail as the pandemic raged out of control, Joe Biden was declared president-elect of the United States. That evening, Biden gave a speech to the nation in which he pledged to make addressing the pandemic his top priority. The next day, Sunday, November 8, the country surpassed its 10 millionth recorded case and was on a clip to add a million more per week—a figure that implied 13,000 deaths per week. In fact, that number would grow to 20,000 weekly deaths by the last week of Trump's presidency.[1]

That same day I received a call from a contact at the Trump White House offering to assist the incoming president's transition team with the pandemic. This was a hopeful sign. But it was not to happen. Rather than worry about the public welfare, President Trump did not concede and instead waged a historic war on the election results, thereby holding up the start of the formal transition process. It would take weeks before the two administrations were permitted to communicate, because although hospitals across the country were overflowing with COVID-19 patients, Trump's own political fight was more important to him. When the outgoing administration finally began to assist with the transition, the help was spare: the Biden team was shown no pandemic playbook, no vaccine distribution plan, no strategies for how to reduce the death toll.

As early as February 2020, Trump's campaign team had warned him that COVID-19 could cost him the election if he didn't address it. He dismissed the idea, just as he dismissed the virus. He did everything he could to publicly minimize the apparent impact of the virus, yet each of those actions only magnified its real impact. As a result, the devastation wrought by the virus will be a significant part of Trump's legacy—and his team's.

On November 30, Scott Atlas resigned from his post as White House scientific advisor. Only weeks later, evidence of the virus's mutation and the reinfections of people who thought they had immunity emerged—an outgrowth of the shameful policies Atlas championed. In December, Deborah Birx decided to retire from government soon after being criticized for traveling to host a Thanksgiving gathering with three generations of family, seeming to ignore the precautions she had urged the rest of the country to observe.

Meanwhile, Bright, Messonnier, Marks, and Fauci were embraced by the Biden administration and asked to play prominent roles.

With life still nowhere close to normal, Lana and I began preparing for a more low-key life as empty-nesters, putting our Minneapolis house on the market and house hunting in her home state of California. But our plans were once again disrupted. In late December, I received a call from Jeff Zients, whom Biden had named to lead the White House's coronavirus response effort. Jeff and I had worked closely together on the successful Healthcare .gov turnaround during the Obama years, the same period in which Ron Klain was leading the Ebola response. Naming Klain as White House chief of staff and Zients as head of the pandemic response were two of the smartest decisions then president-elect Biden could have made. They are both proven, experienced hands, universally respected, and battle-tested. Like others joining the new administration, they are also low-ego, high-integrity human beings who bring both steadiness and aggressiveness to this work.

Zients asked if I would join him, Klain, Fauci, new CDC director Dr. Rochelle Walensky, Dr. David Kessler, and others as part of a team to lead the country's way out of the crisis. I had been resistant to earlier feelers about joining the administration. I found this request more challenging to dismiss. It was an opportunity to serve the country again at a time of need. To make the decision easier, they offered me the opportunity to join for about four months, or through the end of May. It felt like the right amount of time to make a difference and the maximum period I felt I could be away from Lana. What caused me to take the leap was the chance to address the most important challenge that emerged when writing this book: Was our society still capable of working together to solve big problems and define a shared future? The opportunity to be part of turning the page on everything I felt had been so wrong in Trump's handling of the COVID-19 response felt like destiny. Luckily, Lana agreed. So I ditched the sweatpants, packed some suits and ties and shirts into a couple of suitcases, and prepared to reenter the all-consuming world of Washington and the pandemic response.

I arrived in D.C. in mid-January, a couple of days before the inauguration. In my first few meetings, I saw up close the state of the pandemic response we were inheriting. Despite cases and deaths near all-time highs, the vaccination program was woefully behind what the Trump administration had promised, and while the public was growing impatient, there was no plan to change course. Trump's vaccine distribution was rolling out the same way everything else had during the pandemic—designed to minimize political risk—and thereby minimizing results. The public had been lied to and let down to the point where fatigue was high and trust was gone. And the country was no less divided after the election than before. Meanwhile, what Bill Joy had warned me about almost a year before, something that had seemed fanciful at the time, was really happening: dangerous mutations of the virus were popping up in different parts of the world and here in the United States. Every person we didn't vaccinate and every day wasted meant more people would die. Zach's math dictated that the impact of success or failure would be compounded. We had to make a big difference in this response in a short timeframe.

All of this meant we would need to reverse one of Trump's key tenets and begin to assume federal accountability for a crisis in process. The Trump team had set things up so the states were fully responsible for getting people vaccinated and could be blamed when they weren't. It was a self-fulfilling prophecy. Less than half of the vaccines that were delivered were making their way into the arms of people who needed them—the rest were sitting around in the states unused. We quickly enlisted FEMA to set up large-scale vaccination sites and brought in thousands of military servicemen and women to vaccinate the public. By stepping up in that way, more than 75 percent of the vaccines delivered were in use almost immediately, and we soon tripled the daily vaccination rates.

There was no way out of the pandemic without restoring public trust in government. After all, people had to decide whether to take a brand-new vaccine. The clinical trials had shown almost unheard-of results, but only 40 percent of the public said they wanted it, not nearly enough to defeat the virus. Trump's continued promises that the virus would soon magically end had destroyed public trust in government. Soon after the Inauguration, I took the assignment of helping to win back public trust, a mission of extreme importance to President Biden. Taking my cue from him, and from my work over the past year, I looked for the best way to level with the public and restore the independent voice of scientists through a regular communication process.

Trump's press conferences had been a mess—filled with improvisations, bogus science, and lies. A week after the inauguration, I decided to host televised briefings with Tony Fauci and Rochelle Walensky every Monday, Wednesday, and Friday. Before walking out on the stage for the first time to face the cameras, I called Lana for advice. "Competence," she said. "Just show the country some competence."

Three times per week we provided clear, consistent public health messages; honest scientific analysis that covered the good and the bad; and accountability for what we promised to deliver on. We did what everyone says they do, but few actually do: we under-promised and over-delivered on how we would vaccinate the country. The public noticed: the straight talk, the scientific open-book, and the consistent messages contributed to high public approval ratings for Biden's handling of the pandemic. More importantly, surveys showed that trust in the vaccine also increased significantly as people saw the results and began to believe what they heard once again.

Not all the signs were positive. As hospitalizations and deaths from COVID-19 began to diminish, the country was naturally eager to return to the lives and livelihoods they missed. Some couldn't wait for the vaccination efforts to take hold. In early March, Texas eliminated the mandate to wear masks in public settings—despite being next to last in vaccinations, with not even 10 percent of their population vaccinated. Facebook was a large source of misinformation about the vaccines, with posts of giant needles and falsehoods about side effects.

Racism and inequality were two of the most stubborn problems we faced, and they showed up everywhere as we administered vaccinations. As soon as vaccines became available, white suburban populations swooped into hard-hit Black and brown neighborhoods to get the first vaccines, often shutting more at-risk recipients out of appointments.

But something important did change, rather dramatically and with little fanfare. On March 11, the president signed into law the American Rescue Plan, the most far-reaching anti-poverty legislation in a generation. Among many other things, it provided a guaranteed income to every poor and middle-class family in the country, effectively reducing child poverty by half. This meant millions of parents would soon be able to afford to work and care for their children, begin to provide reliable food and shelter for their families, and live with less fear that a single misfortune—big or small—could derail it all.

The legislation and the anti-poverty features were popular with people across the country. It would have been a storybook moment for the country, demonstrating all that had been learned in a year wrestling with a pandemic, but for two things: a number of the measures were only temporary, and, despite being wildly popular with Democrats and Republicans, not a single Republican member of Congress voted for it.

Nevertheless, as our efforts at a competent, honest response continued from the White House, I could feel some of the confidence in our country begin to return. The United States, far and away the leader in deaths from COVID-19, was now far and away the leader in vaccinations. And we began to lead the effort to vaccinate the world, contributing billions of dollars and know-how to vaccinate people in other countries and build new vaccine factories around the world.

Just as many begin to see a light at the end of the tunnel, I can only wonder if the lessons of the past year might be forgotten as security and prosperity return to the country. I hope not. There is so much work to do.

APPENDIX

Exhibit N

Our health care system

We should simplify, reduce costs, and reform step-by-step until the system works for us.

- Insurance is tied to existence, not employment.
- Patients have direct relationships with health care provider groups, not with insurance companies.
- Required investments are made in assisted living facilities.
- A National Institutes of Health Center is created for studying and treating long-term symptoms of COVID-19 and other viruses.
- Required reporting on racial and income disparities is regularly filed and resulting payment changes are made.
- All payer per capita payments to doctors and hospitals are at reasonable levels of margin.
- Progress in health outcomes is measured by analyzing the gap between best and worst care as opposed to simply the average between them.
- Private-sector innovation is centered on the most vulnerable populations.
- A focus on fiscal sustainability is made through scoreable pay-fors and incentives to provide better care for lower costs.

Our safety net

We must give people the freedom from worry and the ability to stay healthy and protect their communities.

- Income support for Americans with children who are experiencing homelessness.
- Every worker has paid medical leave.
- Medicaid increases automatically with unemployment.
- Every unemployed worker receives relief in states of emergency.
- Every small business is protected from interruption.
- We make investments in affordable housing.

Our investments in and reorientation of public health

We should develop the capabilities needed against any enemy: infrastructure, education, and surveillance are key to prevention and a fast start.

- Replenish the National Strategic Stockpile with PPE and medicines.
- Create domestic production of critical medications and a critical health infrastructure.
- Establish biological threat-preparedness positions at the federal (cabinet), state, and municipal levels.
- Require federal, state, and municipal biological response drills every six months.

- The CDC and OSHA create new workplace safety centers targeting infectious diseases.
- Develop diagnostic testing centers of excellence to create rapidly deployable diagnostic testing and genomic sequencing.
- The U.S. distributes masks and makes them readily available for seasonal exposure.
- The Institute of Medicine leads a nonpartisan task force to recommend reforms to the CDC and FDA.
- Paid isolation is available to those infected with or exposed to COVID-19.
- The U.S. participates in global antiviral and vaccine research.
- The CDC conducts national weekly briefings and color-code updating.
- Public health is included in curricula beginning in elementary school.
- A full-time public health service corps for contact tracing is created.
- The U.S. develops a public health surveillance response and alert communication system like the national weather service.
- We elevate patient and caregiver voices in policymaking.

Our pandemic response

We need to build and exercise the muscles to make the response to a pandemic easier on everyone.

- Vaccinations will be free.
- We will have national color-coded criteria for shutting down and opening up, to be implemented community by community.
- We will establish centers for testing and mask distribution.
- We will create hub-and-spoke public health and infectious disease centers.
- There will be a process in place for airport and transportation hub quarantining.
- There will be a Biological Response Command Center.
- We will establish an Epidemiology Containment Unit Response program.

Congressional and legal response

We need Congress to provide checks and balances, investments, and more authority.

- Mandatory public health measures will be allowed in approved states of emergency, recommended by the CDC and requiring continual reauthorization by Congress.
- Funding for the NIH, BARDA, CDC, and FDA will be increased and tied to reforms.
- Congress will have oversight authority over the Executive Branch biological threat response.

Social underpinnings

We won't really fix things until . . .

- we have voting reforms;
- we pass lobbying reforms;
- scientific institutions have a high degree of independence from political interference;
- we have nationwide broadband;
- everyone is paid a living wage;
- everyone has affordable housing;
- inequality is addressed through the tax code and other policy initiatives.

ACKNOWLEDGMENTS

It was challenging to write a book about an event that included the loss of so many people while still respecting how personal each loss was to those left behind. As the death toll mounted, there were nights when I was writing this that it was difficult to feel the most recent deaths as deeply as the first. I really wanted to get this right, and I know I will regret all the times when I didn't properly account for what happened. From the very beginning of the pandemic, I had friends who lost loved ones, right up until the day I turned the book in, when a close friend lost his father-in-law. For the several million other people who lost a parent, child, sibling, grandparent, spouse, or friend, I wanted this story told so your grief could be tied to a record of events. I had to write parts of this book over and over to try to accomplish this. Having never written a book before, and wanting it to be a good book, I was willing to take all the help I could get. And the people who helped me were generous and gifted. It is important that I name them and their role in creating this book.

To current and former FDA, HHS, NIH, NIAID, BARDA, White House, CDC, and WHO officials who made sure this story was true not just at a high level, but also in the subtleties, I am grateful. I want to thank the many people who told me their stories; I tried to include those whose experiences were as representative of the country's experience as possible. If your story wasn't included, I hope its essence is captured in the stories of Cleavon Gilman, Thia, Melissa, and Ahmed. (Cleavon's last name is real; for the others, some parts of their names were modified.) Hopefully you feel more seen. I regretfully cut an entire chapter about the many people who did so much for others during this challenging time—from Chef José Andrés and his World Central Kitchen to the team behind the open-source low-cost Saliva Direct test, to Andrew Stroup's Project N95, which sourced crucial PPE, and to the people at United States of Care who turned on a dime to provide critical support and information to state governments. To the other people in this book whose stories I told, in particular, Blythe Adamson, Rick Bright, Larry Brilliant, John Doerr, Baruch Fischhoff, Corey Johnson, Bill Joy, Peter Marks, Nancy Messonnier, Mike Osterholm, and Ryan Panchadsaram, to name a few, I hope I correctly captured your work and contributions.

So many people helped me write this book. My research assistant, Nath Samaratunga, is a graduate student in public health, and soon to enter medical school. He researched every fact, found every piece of data, found great information I was missing, confirmed or corrected data, and that was just his day job. He also read and reread what I wrote, and made it better. He made sure I was true to every person whose story I told, and he shared his opinions with me continually. He told me what was good and what needed work. My name is on the cover but this is our work together, Nath. In addition, my first research assistant, Sara Lederman, a medical student with a master's degree in public health, provided vital help as I began this book. She relished hearing and capturing people's stories. If what's missing in this world is empathy, Sara is the cure.

To everyone who reviewed pieces of the book, including David Agus, Richard Frank, Vikki Wachino, Niall Brennan, Eli Casdin, and several anonymous people in the Trump administration, thank you. The many scientists who informed this effort include David Agus, Nahid Bhadelia, Larry Brilliant, Rob Califf, Baruch Fischhoff, Tom Frieden, Laurie Garrett, Atul Gawande, Scott Gottlieb, Bill Joy, Mark McClellan, Mike Osterholm, Angela Rasmussen, Caitlin Rivers, Leana Wen, and Ed Yong. Not only are they some of our best scientific minds, they turned out to be great human beings as well.

The people at the publishing house were good editors, but there was no more thorough editor than my wife, Lana. You challenged me to make my point clearer over and over and called BS when you read something that was too much my version of events. I loved when you just wrote "meh" next to some anecdote I was trying to tell. My entire childhood my dad brandished his red pen on every single thing I wrote. I mean, there wasn't a single sentence that escaped his corrections and improvements. I don't know what he would have thought of this book, but he would have approved of Lana's editing job. "Not bad," he would have said.

When the publisher suggested I consider working with an editor, I didn't realize how much a great one like Matt Sharpe could help. He was gracious but unsparing. There were many parts of this book cut. They were fun to write, good stories, and a large part of what I lived, but Matt told me when they didn't belong. And he was invariably right.

At St. Martin's Press, I got the A-team. Tim Bartlett took over this project as executive editor from Stephen Power. Stephen was incredibly encouraging. He helped me spin up ideas, and the book wouldn't be here without him. When Tim took over the project, he was detailed and specific with his feedback, and I grew to crave his critiques. He thought for the reader at every moment and pushed me to reveal what really mattered. The contributions of Alan Bradshaw, Laura Clark, Alice Pfeifer, and Sue Warga made the book better. Gabrielle Gantz, Tracey Guest, Rob Grom, Meryl Sussman Levavi, and Daniel Prielipp turned this into a finished product.

The gifts from my parents are not fixed, but have been given to evolve to find me at each stage. I learned to listen with empathy from my mother, Beth, which was essential in writing this book. My father, Earl, showed me how to find poetry in the most humble acts of kindness, service, and effort. I am grateful for the encouragement, love, and support that my siblings, Lesley and Gabriel, showed me during the process and always.

To my sons, as I said to you every night while tucking you into bed as little boys, Caleb, you're the greatest, and Zach, you're the best. Your mom and I are so proud of the young men you've grown into and hope that you will continue to demonstrate empathy and kindness to those around you. Your biggest regrets will be the times when you don't. And to my wife, Lana, you always say you're my number one fan. I hope you know I'm your number one fan too.

NOTES

Preface

1. World Health Organization, "WHO Coronavirus (COVID-19) Dashboard," https://covid19.who.int/?gclid=CjwKCAiAg8OBBhA8EiwAlKw3kr8w-eQa -SmMo8RvcoXQhJKmYxSUu1Q16NddY_2BTm5wKrQ7w6uZnoRoCE -CYQAvD_BwE.

Introduction

1. Andy Slavitt, "Currently experts expect over 1 million deaths in the U.S. since the virus was not contained & we cannot even test for it. This will be recorded as a major preventable public health disaster. I will try to relate what I learned from a long day of calls about what is happening," Twitter, March 12, 2020, 11:18 p.m., https://twitter.com/ASlavitt/status/1238303395448008704.
2. "Our Data," COVID Tracking Project, accessed September 27, 2020, https://covidtracking.com/data.
3. "Why 'Exponential Growth' Is So Scary for the COVID-19 Coronavirus," *Forbes*, March 17, 2020, https://www.forbes.com/sites/startswithabang/2020/03/17/why-exponential-growth-is-so-scary-for-the-covid-19-coronavirus/#17def89b4e9b.
4. Steve Eder, Henry Fountain, Michael H. Keller, Muyi Xiao, and Alexandra Stevenson, "430,000 People Have Traveled from China to U.S. Since Coronavirus Surfaced," *New York Times*, April 15, 2020, https://www.nytimes.com/2020/04/04/us/coronavirus-china-travel-restrictions.html.

5. David Leonhardt, "America's Death Gap," *New York Times*, September 1, 2020, https://www.nytimes.com/2020/09/01/briefing/coronavirus-kenosha-massachusetts-your-tuesday-briefing.html.

6. Peter Mwai, "Coronavirus: Is the Rate of Growth in Africa Slowing Down?," *BBC News*, September 25, 2020, https://www.bbc.com/news/world-africa-53181555.

7. Fiona M. Guerra et al., "The Basic Reproduction Number (R0) of Measles: A Systematic Review," *Lancet Infectious Diseases* 17, no. 12 (July 27, 2017): e420–28, https://doi.org/10.1016/s1473–3099(17)30307–9.

Chapter 1: Is This Really Happening?

1. "Remarks by President Trump in Press Conference 2.25.20," The White House, February 25, 2020, https://www.whitehouse.gov/briefings-statements/remarks-president-trump-press-conference-4.

2. Justin Wise, "Kudlow Claims Coronavirus Has Been Contained: 'It's Pretty Close to Air-Tight,'" *The Hill*, February 25, 2020, https://thehill.com/homenews/administration/484561-kudlow-claims-coronavirus-has-been-contained-its-pretty-close-to-air.

3. James Griffiths, "Coronavirus Deaths Top 2,200 as Number of New Cases Rises Again," CNN, February 21, 2020, https://www.cnn.com/2020/02/21/asia/novel-coronavirus-covid-19-update-intl-hnk/index.html.

4. "Mini-Episode: Andy Calls CBS Correspondent Seth Doane in Rome," *In the Bubble with Andy Slavitt*, April 11, 2020, https://www.lemonadamedia.com/podcast/mini-episode-seth-doane.

5. Joe Hasell, "Testing Early, Testing Late: Four Countries' Approaches to COVID-19 Testing Compared," Our World in Data, May 19, 2020, https://ourworldindata.org/covid-testing-us-uk-korea-italy.

6. Hasell, "Testing Early, Testing Late."

7. "NHE Fact Sheet," Centers for Medicare and Medicaid Services, accessed February 23, 2020, https://www.cms.gov/research-statistics-data-and-systems/statistics-trends-and-reports/nationalhealthexpenddata/nhe-fact-sheet.

8. Katie Young, "Need for Nurses Is Driving Record Pay as Coronavirus Nears Its Peak," CNBC, April 2, 2020, https://www.cnbc.com/2020/04/02/need-for-nurses-is-driving-record-pay-as-coronavirus-nears-its-peak.html.

9. "Find the Helpers," *In the Bubble with Andy Slavitt*, April 1, 2020, https://www.lemonadamedia.com/podcast/in-the-bubble-find-the-helpers.

10. Ricky O'Donnell, "The NBA Suspends Season over Coronavirus Pandemic," SBNation.com, March 11, 2020, https://www.sbnation.com/2020/3/11/21175978/nba-season-suspended-coronavirus-pandemic-rudy-gobert.

11. Caroline Kelly, "Rep. Matt Gaetz Wore a Gas Mask on House Floor During Vote on Coronavirus Response Package," CNN, updated March 9, 2020,

https://www.cnn.com/2020/03/04/politics/gaetz-coronavirus-gas-mask/index
.html.

12. "Public Health Officials Report Florida's First 2 COVID-19 Deaths," last
updated March 7, 2020, https://www.local10.com/news/local/2020/03/07/2
-florida-covid-19-patients-die-public-health-officials-say.

13. "'I Shook Hands with Everybody,' Says Boris Johnson Weeks Before Coronavirus Diagnosis," *Guardian*, March 27, 2020, https://www.theguardian
.com/world/video/2020/mar/27/i-shook-hands-with-everybody-says-boris
-johnson-weeks-before-coronavirus-diagnosis-video.

14. Greg Newkirk, "They deleted the tweet this morning, but it's still appearing if
you click through from a link. Less than a month ago Herman Cain tweeted
this. He died from COVID-19 this morning," Twitter, July 30, 2020, 11:24
a.m., https://twitter.com/nuekerk/status/1288858078700593152.

15. Andy Slavitt, "COVID-19 Prep Update—March 14," Twitter, March 14,
2020, 9:20 a.m., https://twitter.com/ASlavitt/status/1238817274590629888.

16. Jeff Zillgit, "Coronavirus: NBA Star Karl-Anthony Towns Loses Mom to
COVID-19," *USA Today*, April 13, 2020, https://www.usatoday.com/story
/sports/nba/twolves/2020/04/13/mother-timberwolves-karl-anthony-towns
-dies-coronavirus/2984903001.

17. "Mini-Episode: Andy Calls Senator Amy Klobuchar," *In the Bubble with
Andy Slavitt*, April 4, 2020, https://www.lemonadamedia.com/podcast/bubble
-klobuchar.

18. WDIV (Detroit), "President Trump, Michigan Gov. Whitmer Spar over Supply Shortage amid COVID-19 Outbreak," YouTube, posted March 27, 2020,
https://www.youtube.com/watch?v=UmugGJW3mWo.

19. "Find the Helpers," *In the Bubble with Andy Slavitt*, https://www.lemonadamedia
.com/show/in-the-bubble, April 1, 2020.

20. "Find the Helpers."

21. Apoorva Mandavilli, "Even Asymptomatic People Carry the Coronavirus in
High Amounts," *New York Times*, August 6, 2020, https://www.nytimes.com
/2020/08/06/health/coronavirus-asymptomatic-transmission.html.

22. Christie Aschwanden, "How 'Superspreading' Events Drive Most COVID-19
Spread," *Scientific American*, June 23, 2020, https://www.scientificamerican
.com/article/how-superspreading-events-drive-most-covid-19-spread1.

23. Kai Kupferschmidt, "Why Do Some COVID-19 Patients Infect Many Others,
Whereas Most Don't Spread the Virus at All?," *Science*, May 19, 2020, https://
www.sciencemag.org/news/2020/05/why-do-some-covid-19-patients-infect
-many-others-whereas-most-don-t-spread-virus-all.

24. "What Is Known About COVID-19 and Abnormal Blood Clotting," press
release, Weill Cornell Medicine, July 2, 2020, https://news.weill.cornell.edu
/news/2020/07/what-is-known-about-covid-19-and-abnormal-blood-clotting.

25. "Why COVID-19 Makes Some People So Much Sicker Than Others," Yale Medicine, April 9, 2020, https://www.yalemedicine.org/stories/immune-response-covid-19.

26. "COVID-19: Who's at Higher Risk of Serious Symptoms?," Mayo Clinic, August 21, 2020, https://www.mayoclinic.org/diseases-conditions/coronavirus/in-depth/coronavirus-who-is-at-risk/art-20483301.

27. "Spread and Transmission," Coronavirus.gov, accessed October 1, 2020, https://faq.coronavirus.gov/spread-transmission.

28. Ricardo Alonso-Zaldivar, "Nursing Home COVID-19 Cases Rise Four-Fold in Surge States," Associated Press, November 8, 2020, https://apnews.com/article/virus-outbreak-only-on-ap-chicago-nursing-homes-596ef4bfe18313ae72368e2c86e85f27.

29. Denise Grady, "Fauci Warns That the Coronavirus Pandemic Is Far from Over," *New York Times*, June 9, 2020, https://www.nytimes.com/2020/06/09/health/fauci-vaccines-coronavirus.html.

30. Stephanie Soucheray, "Osterholm Plays Detective, General in 'Deadliest Enemy' Book," Center for Infectious Disease Research and Policy, University of Minnesota, March 14, 2020, https://www.cidrap.umn.edu/news-perspective/2017/03/osterholm-plays-detective-general-deadliest-enemy-book.

31. Michael T. Osterholm et al., "My Views on Cloth Face Coverings for the Public for Preventing COVID-19," Center for Infectious Disease Research and Policy, University of Minnesota, July 22, 2020, https://www.cidrap.umn.edu/news-perspective/2020/07/commentary-my-views-cloth-face-coverings-public-preventing-covid-19.

32. Peter Bergen, "Michael Osterholm: Infectious Disease Expert Says We're Only in the Second Inning of the Pandemic," CNN, April 21, 2020, https://www.cnn.com/2020/04/21/opinions/bergen-osterholm-interview-two-opinion/index.html.

33. Bergen, "Michael Osterholm: Infectious Disease Expert Says"; "CIDRAP Covid-19 Viewpoint Part 1," Center for Infectious Disease Research and Policy, University of Minnesota, April 30, 2020, https://www.cidrap.umn.edu/sites/default/files/public/downloads/cidrap-covid19-viewpoint-part1_0.pdf.

34. Apoorva Mandavilli, "Covid-19: What if 'Herd Immunity' Is Closer Than Scientists Thought?," *New York Times*, August 17, 2020, https://www.nytimes.com/2020/08/17/health/coronavirus-herd-immunity.html; Sarah Boseley, "Coronavirus 'Could Infect 60 Percent of Global Population if Unchecked,'" *Guardian*, February 11, 2020, https://www.theguardian.com/world/2020/feb/11/coronavirus-expert-warns-infection-could-reach-60-of-worlds-population.

35. "Emergencies Preparedness, Response, 2020," World Health Organization, accessed October 11, 2020, http://www.who.int/csr/don/archive/year/2020/en.

36. "Global Health Observatory," World Health Organization, accessed October 11, 2020, https://www.who.int/data/gho; "Number of Deaths Due to Cholera," World Health Organization, accessed October 11, 2020, https://www.who.int /gho/epidemic_diseases/cholera/situation_trends_deaths/en; "2009 H1N1 Pandemic," Centers for Disease Control and Prevention, June 11, 2019, https:// www.cdc.gov/flu/pandemic-resources/2009-h1n1-pandemic.html.

37. "Hong Kong: Novel Coronavirus Development 2020," Statista, accessed November 9, 2020, https://www.statista.com/statistics/1105425/hong-kong -novel-coronavirus-covid19-confirmed-death-recovered-trend.

38. Zeynep Tufekci, "How Hong Kong Is Beating the Coronavirus," *The Atlantic*, May 12, 2020, https://www.theatlantic.com/technology/archive/2020/05/how -hong-kong-beating-coronavirus/611524.

39. COVID Tracking Project, "Our Data," accessed September 27, 2020, https:// covidtracking.com/data.

40. COVID Tracking Project, "Our Data"; Alexei Koseff, "Gov. Gavin Newsom Ramps Up California's Response to the Coronavirus," *San Francisco Chronicle*, March 13, 2020, https://www.sfchronicle.com/politics/article/Newsom -ramps-up-California-s-response-to-the-15127288.php.

41. COVID Tracking Project, "Our Data."

42. John Commins, "Study Puts U.S. COVID-19 Infection Fatality Rate at 1.3 Percent," HealthLeaders, May 7, 2020, https://www.healthleadersmedia.com /covid-19/study-puts-us-covid-19-infection-fatality-rate-13.

43. Andy Slavitt, "We have learned the daunting power of exponential math when it comes to infection rate or R0," Twitter, April 25, 2020, 11:11 p.m., https://twitter.com/aslavitt/status/1254246666686922752?lang=en.

44. Lauren Egan, "Trump Calls Coronavirus Democrats' 'New Hoax,'" NBC News, February 28, 2020, https://www.nbcnews.com/politics/donald-trump /trump-calls-coronavirus-democrats-new-hoax-n1145721.

45. "Andy Slavitt: Slowing Spread of Coronavirus 'Is in Our Hands,'" *Kasie DC*, MSNBC, March 19, 2020, https://www.msnbc.com/kasie-dc/watch/andy -slavitt-slowing-spread-of-coronavirus-is-in-our-hands-81359429764.

Chapter 2: Unexploded Bombs

1. "Health Insurance Coverage of the Total Population," KFF, accessed October 11, 2020, https://www.kff.org/other/state-indicator/total-population /?currentTimeframe.

2. Morgan Haefner, "Cancer Forces 42 Percent of Patients to Exhaust Life Savings in 2 Years, Study Finds," *Becker's Hospital Review*, October 24, 2018, https://www.beckershospitalreview.com/finance/cancer-forces-42-of-patients -to-exhaust-life-savings-in-2-years-study-finds.html.

3. Juliana Menasce Horowitz, Ruth Igielnik, and Rakesh Kochhar, "Trends in U.S. Income and Wealth Inequality," Pew Research Center, Social and Demographic Trends Project, January 9, 2020, https://www.pewsocialtrends.org /2020/01/09/trends-in-income-and-wealth-inequality; Jamie Ducharme and Elijah Wolfson, "How Your Zip Code Could Affect Your Lifespan," *Time*, June 17, 2019, https://time.com/5608268/zip-code-health; "Racial and Ethnic Disparities Continue in Pregnancy-Related Deaths," Centers for Disease Control, September 6, 2019, https://www.cdc.gov/media/releases/2019/p0905 -racial-ethnic-disparities-pregnancy-deaths.html; National Center for Health Statistics, "Health, United States, 2015: With Special Feature on Racial and Ethnic Health Disparities," 2016, https://www.ncbi.nlm.nih.gov/books /NBK367643.

4. "Healthy Futures Summit & SPH 75th Anniversary Gala," School of Public Health, University of Minnesota, December 5, 2019, https://www.sph.umn .edu/events-calendar/healthy-futures-summit.

5. "Mortality in the United States: Past, Present, and Future," Penn Wharton Budget Model, June 27, 2016, https://budgetmodel.wharton.upenn.edu/issues /2016/1/25/mortality-in-the-united-states-past-present-and-future.

6. "The Impact of Chronic Underfunding of America's Public Health System: Trends, Risks, and Recommendations, 2019," Trust for America's Health, April 2019, https://www.tfah.org/report-details/2019-funding-report; "New TFAH Report: Persistent Underfunding of America's Public Health System Makes the Nation Vulnerable and Puts Lives at Risk," Trust for America's Health, April 24, 2019, https://www.tfah.org/article/new-tfah-report -persistent-underfunding-of-americas-public-health-system-makes-the-nation -vulnerable-and-puts-lives-at-risk.

7. Ed Yong, "Why the Pandemic Is So Bad in America," *The Atlantic*, August 4, 2020, https://www.theatlantic.com/magazine/archive/2020/09/coronavirus -american-failure/614191; Jeremy Konyndyk, "American Exceptionalism Failed the Test of the Coronavirus Pandemic," *Foreign Affairs*, June 8, 2020, https:// www.foreignaffairs.com/articles/united-states/2020-06-08/exceptionalism -killing-americans; Trust for America's Health, "New TFAH Report"; Liz Alesse, "Did Trump Try to Cut the CDC's Budget as Democrats Claim?," ABC News, February 28, 2020, https://abcnews.go.com/Politics/trump-cut-cdcs -budget-democrats-claim-analysis/story?id=69233170.

8. "Strategic National Stockpile Fact Sheet," Association of State and Territorial Health Officials, accessed October 11, 2020, https://www.astho.org /Programs/Preparedness/Public-Health-Emergency-Law/Emergency-Use -Authorization-Toolkit/Strategic-National-Stockpile-Fact-Sheet; Beth Reinhard and Emma Brown, "Face Masks in National Stockpile of Medical Supplies Have Not Been Substantially Replenished Since 2009," *Washington*

Post, March 10, 2020, https://www.washingtonpost.com/investigations /face-masks-in-national-stockpile-have-not-been-substantially-replenished -since-2009/2020/03/10/57e57316–60c9–11ea-8baf-519cedb6ccd9_story .html; Yeganeh Torbati and Isaac Arnsdorf, "How Tea Party Budget Battles Left the National Emergency Medical Stockpile Unprepared for Coronavirus," *ProPublica*, April 3, 2020, https://www.propublica.org/article/us-emergency -medical-stockpile-funding-unprepared-coronavirus?token=0ceE -HgXEaOXnSqRQtXN6xdb2ukKaUJw; Noam N. Levy, Kim Christensen, and Anna M. Phillips, "A Disaster Foretold: Shortages of Ventilators and Other Medical Supplies Have Long Been Warned About," *Los Angeles Times*, March 20, 2020, https://www.latimes.com/politics/story/2020–03–20 /disaster-foretold-shortages-ventilators-medical-supplies-warned-about.

9. Victoria Knight, "Obama Team Left Pandemic Playbook for Trump Administration, Officials Confirm," *PBS NewsHour*, May 15, 2020, https://www .pbs.org/newshour/nation/obama-team-left-pandemic-playbook-for-trump -administration-officials-confirm.

10. "Fact Sheet: The Global Health Security Agenda," The White House, July 28, 2015, https://obamawhitehouse.archives.gov/the-press-office/2015/07/28 /fact-sheet-global-health-security-agenda.

11. Deb Riechmann, "Trump Disbanded NSC Pandemic Unit That Experts Had Praised," Associated Press, March 14, 2020, https://apnews.com/article/ce01 4d94b64e98b7203b873e56f80e9a.

12. Nicholas Confessore, "Mick Mulvaney's Master Class in Destroying a Bureaucracy from Within," *New York Times*, April 16, 2019, https://www.nytimes .com/2019/04/16/magazine/consumer-financial-protection-bureau-trump .html; Nadja Popovich, Livia Albeck-Ripka, and Kendra Pierre-Louis, "The Trump Administration Is Reversing 100 Environmental Rules. Here's the Full List," *New York Times*, June 2, 2019, https://www.nytimes.com/interactive /2020/climate/trump-environment-rollbacks.html.

13. Lena H. Sun, "CDC to Cut by 80 Percent Efforts to Prevent Global Disease Outbreak," *Washington Post*, February 1, 2018, https://www.washingtonpost.com /news/to-your-health/wp/2018/02/01/cdc-to-cut-by-80-percent-efforts-to -prevent-global-disease-outbreak; Kim Krisberg, "President's Budget Would Hinder US Public Health Progress: Huge Cuts Proposed," *Nation's Health* 49, no. 3 (May 2019), https://thenationshealth.aphapublications.org/content /49/3/1.2.

14. "Remarks of the President—As Prepared for Delivery—Signing of Stem Cell Executive Order and Scientific Integrity Presidential Memorandum," The White House, March 9, 2009, https://obamawhitehouse.archives.gov/the-press -office/remarks-president-prepared-delivery-signing-stem-cell-executive-order -and-scientifi.

15. Lena H. Sun, "Trump Officials Seek Greater Control over CDC Reports on Coronavirus," *Washington Post*, Sepember 12, 2020, https://www.washingtonpost.com/health/2020/09/12/trump-control-over-cdc-reports.

16. Mike Stobbe, "Health Official Who Urged Abstinence Says Views Have Changed," Associated Press, June 29, 2018, https://apnews.com/article/31efa34661ff48ffa30e488c013640b7.

17. "What No One Knows About COVID-19, with Larry Brilliant," *In the Bubble with Andy Slavitt*, July 22, 2020, https://www.lemonadamedia.com/podcast/what-no-one-knows-about-covid-19-with-larry-brilliant.

18. "KFF Health Tracking Poll—May 2020," KFF, May 27, 2020, https://www.kff.org/coronavirus-covid-19/report/kff-health-tracking-poll-may-2020.

Chapter 3: Waking Up Late

1. Erica Werner, Yasmeen Abutaleb, Lena H. Sun, and Lenny Bernstein, "Trump Officials Warn of Inevitable Spread of Coronavirus Across the United States," *Washington Post*, February 25, 2020, https://www.washingtonpost.com/us-policy/2020/02/25/cdc-coronavirus-inevitable.

2. J. Edward Moreno, "Trump Threatened to Fire CDC's Chief of Respiratory Diseases in February: Report," *The Hill*, April 22, 2020, https://thehill.com/homenews/administration/494187-trump-threatened-to-fire-cdcs-chief-of-respiratory-diseases-in.

3. Werner et al., "Trump Officials Warn of Inevitable Spread."

4. "Transcript: U.S. Health Officials on Response to Coronavirus February 25, 2020," C-SPAN, February 25, 2020, https://www.rev.com/blog/transcripts/transcript-u-s-health-officials-on-response-to-coronavirus-february-25-2020.

5. Bill Chappell, "Trump Often Gives 'Complete Opposite' of Health Experts' Advice, Former Staffer Says," NPR, September 30, 2020, https://www.npr.org/2020/09/30/918333059/trump-often-gives-complete-opposite-of-health-experts-advice-former-staffer-says.

6. Philip Rucker, Laurie McGinley, Josh Dawsey, and Yasmeen Abutaleb, "Rancor Between Scientists and Trump Allies Threatens Pandemic Response as Cases Surge," *Washington Post*, July 17, 2020, https://www.washingtonpost.com/politics/rancor-between-scientists-and-trump-allies-threatens-pandemic-response-as-cases-surge/2020/07/17/d950e9b6-c777-11ea-a99f-3bbdffb1af38_story.html.

7. Dareh Gregorian, "Trump Told Bob Woodward He Knew in February That COVID-19 Was 'Deadly Stuff' but Wanted to 'Play It Down,'" NBC News, September 9, 2020, https://www.nbcnews.com/politics/donald-trump/trump-told-bob-woodward-he-knew-february-covid-19-was-n1239658.

8. Andy Slavitt, "A message to the people who turn to this account for health care politics," Twitter, March 16, 2020, https://twitter.com/aslavitt/status /1239639514823483394?lang=en.

9. Serena Dai, "Alexandria Ocasio-Cortez Implores New Yorkers to Stop Crowding Bars and Restaurants," *Eater NY*, March 14, 2020, https://ny.eater .com/2020/3/14/21179790/coronavirus-nyc-restaurants-alexandria-ocasio -cortez; Chris Cillizza, "Devin Nunes' Outrageous Explanation for His Coronavirus Comments," CNN, March 17, 2020, https://www.cnn.com/2020/03 /17/politics/devin-nunes-hannity-coronavirus/index.html.

10. "Mini-Episode: Our First 50-State Emergency (with Juliette Kayyem)," *In the Bubble with Andy Slavitt*, April 27, 2020, https://www.lemonadamedia.com /podcast/in-the-bubble-juliette-kayyem.

11. Peter Bergen, "Infectious Disease Expert: We're Only in the Second Inning of the Pandemic," CNN, April 22, 2020, https://www.cnn.com/2020/04/21 /opinions/bergen-osterholm-interview-two-opinion/index.html.

12. Tom Frieden, "Could Coronavirus Kill a Million Americans?," Think Global Health, March 10, 2020, https://www.thinkglobalhealth.org/article/could -coronavirus-kill-million-americans.

13. Lori Robertson, "Trump's Snowballing China Travel Claim," FactCheck.org, April 10, 2020, https://www.factcheck.org/2020/04/trumps-snowballing-china -travel-claim.

14. J. M. Rieger, "The Number of Lives Trump Claims He Has Saved from Covid-19 Has Swelled as the Death Toll Has Grown," *Washington Post*, July 29, 2020, https://www.washingtonpost.com/politics/2020/07/29/number-lives -trump-claims-he-has-saved-covid-19-has-swelled-death-toll-has-grown.

15. Steve Eder, Henry Fountain, Michael H. Keller, Muyi Xiao, and Alexandra Stevenson, "430,000 People Have Traveled from China to U.S. Since Coronavirus Surfaced," *New York Times*, April 4, 2020, https://www.nytimes.com /2020/04/04/us/coronavirus-china-travel-restrictions.html.

16. Carl Zimmer, "Most New York Coronavirus Cases Came from Europe, Genomes Show," *New York Times*, April 8, 2020, https://www.nytimes.com/2020 /04/08/science/new-york-coronavirus-cases-europe-genomes.html.

17. Andy Slavitt, "Currently experts expect over 1 million deaths in the U.S. since the virus was not contained & we cannot even test for it," Twitter, March 12, 2020, 11:18 p.m., https://twitter.com/ASlavitt/status/1238303395448008704.

18. "Bill Joy: What I'm Worried About, What I'm Excited About," TED Talk, February 2006, https://www.ted.com/talks/bill_joy_what_i_m_worried_about _what_i_m_excited_about/transcript.

19. Javier C. Hernández, "After New Coronavirus Outbreaks, China Imposes Wuhan-Style Lockdown," *New York Times*, June 17, 2020, https://www .nytimes.com/2020/05/21/world/asia/coronavirus-china-lockdown.html.

20. Steve Kashkett, "Czech Government Implemented a Face Mask Requirement to Help Combat Covid-19," *USA Today*, April 4, 2020, https://www.usatoday .com/story/opinion/2020/04/04/czech-government-implemented-face-mask -requirement-help-combat-coronavirus-column/2940393001.

21. "Penalties Hiked for COVID-19 Rule Violators in Greece, No Prosecutions Reported," *National Herald*, June 19, 2020, https://www.thenationalherald .com/greece_economy/arthro/penalties_hiked_for_covid_19_rule_violators _in_greece_no_prosecutions_reported-469339.

22. Mark Wilson, "To Stomp Out COVID-19, America Needs a Better Warning System," *Fast Company*, April 6, 2020, https://www.fastcompany.com /90485589/to-stomp-out-covid-19-america-will-need-a-better-warning -system.

23. Saskia Miller, "Angela Merkel's Scientific Background Could Save Germany," *The Atlantic*, April 20, 2020, https://www.theatlantic.com/international /archive/2020/04/angela-merkel-germany-coronavirus-pandemic/610225.

24. Noelle J. Molé, "Trusted Puppets, Tarnished Politicians: Humor and Cynicism in Berlusconi's Italy," *American Ethnologist* 40, no. 2 (May 2013): 288–99, https://doi.org/10.1111/amet.12021.

25. "The Best Thing Everyday Americans Can Do to Fight Coronavirus? #Stay-Home, Save Lives," *USA Today*, March 15, 2020, https://www.usatoday.com /story/opinion/2020/03/15/coronavirus-stay-home-hel-america-save-lives -column/5054241002.

26. "Governor Gavin Newsom Issues Stay at Home Order," Office of Governor Gavin Newsom, March 19, 2020, https://www.gov.ca.gov/2020/03/19 /governor-gavin-newsom-issues-stay-at-home-order.

27. Sarah Mervosh, Denise Lu, and Vanessa Swales, "See Which States and Cities Have Told Residents to Stay at Home," *New York Times*, last updated April 20, 2020, https://www.nytimes.com/interactive/2020/us/coronavirus-stay-at -home-order.html.

28. Kevin Systrom and Thomas Vladec, "R_t COVID-19," accessed October 31, 2020, https://rt.live.

29. Solomon Hsiang et al., "The Effect of Large-Scale Anti-Contagion Policies on the COVID-19 Pandemic," *Nature* 584, no. 7820 (August 2020): 262–67, https://doi.org/10.1038/s41586-020-2404-8.

30. Peter Dizikes, "The Data Speak: Stronger Pandemic Response Yields Better Economic Recovery," press release, Massachusetts Institute of Technology, March 31, 2020, https://news.mit.edu/2020/pandemic-health-response -economic-recovery-0401.

31. Eliza Forsythe et al., "Labor Demand in the Time of COVID-19: Evidence from Vacancy Postings and UI Claims," Working Paper 27061, National Bureau of Economic Research, April 2020, https://doi.org/10.3386/w27061.

32. Yen Nee Lee, "These Asian Economies Seem to Have Contained the Coronavirus Outbreak. Here's How They Did It," CNBC, May 19, 2020, https://www.cnbc.com/2020/05/19/how-taiwan-hong-kong-vietnam-contain-the-coronavirus-outbreak.html; Martin Farrer, "New Zealand's Covid-19 Response the Best in the World, Say Global Business Leaders," *Guardian*, October 7, 2020, https://www.theguardian.com/world/2020/oct/08/new-zealands-covid-19-response-the-best-in-the-world-say-global-business-leaders.

33. Andy Slavitt, "As we cross the 100 death mark today," Twitter, March 17, 2020, https://twitter.com/aslavitt/status/1240063693028810752.

34. "Mini-Episode: Slavitt and Scaramucci Unfiltered," *In the Bubble with Andy Slavitt*, April 20, 2020, https://www.lemonadamedia.com/podcast/in-the-bubble-scaramucci.

35. "Remarks by President Trump, Vice President Pence, and Members of the Coronavirus Task Force in Press Briefing," The White House, March 17, 2020, https://www.whitehouse.gov/briefings-statements/remarks-president-trump-vice-president-pence-members-coronavirus-task-force-press-briefing-4.

Chapter 4: The Virus and the White House, Part I

1. World Health Organization, "WHO Transcript, Emergencies Coronavirus Press Conference, Full," March 13, 2020, https://www.who.int/docs/default-source/coronaviruse/transcripts/who-transcript-emergencies-coronavirus-press-conference-full-13mar2020848c48d2065143bd8d07a1647c863d6b.pdf?sfvrsn=23dd0b04_2.

2. Heungsup Sung et al., "Preparedness and Rapid Implementation of External Quality Assessment Helped Quickly Increase COVID-19 Testing Capacity in the Republic of Korea," *Clinical Chemistry* 66, no. 7 (July 2020): 979–81, https://doi.org/10.1093/clinchem/hvaa097.

3. Atul Gawande, "We Can Solve the Coronavirus-Test Mess Now—If We Want To," *New Yorker*, September 2, 2020, https://www.newyorker.com/science/medical-dispatch/we-can-solve-the-coronavirus-test-mess-now-if-we-want-to.

4. Caroline Chen, Marshall Allen, Lexi Churchill, and Isaac Arnsdorf, "Key Missteps at the CDC Have Set Back Its Ability to Detect the Potential Spread of Coronavirus," *ProPublica*, February 28, 2020, https://www.propublica.org/article/cdc-coronavirus-covid-19-test?token=jg6nGk6aRoymOqJmDTSthj1PIBKaGEW9.

5. Victor Garcia, "Pence Updates Coronavirus Response, Says There Will Be 'Tens of Thousands of Tests' in Coming Days, Weeks," Fox News, March 17, 2020, https://www.foxnews.com/media/mike-pence-coronavirus-response-thousands-tests.

6. Caitlin Owens, "Inside the Bitter Feud at Trump's Health Agencies," *Axios*, December 18, 2019, https://www.axios.com/hhs-azar-verma-feud-45765800-f6d5-4f26-bf76-8f19ab1a8a0a.html.

7. Dan Diamond, Adam Cancryn, and Rachana Pradhan, "Azar, Verma Battle for Trump's Favor amid White House Showdown," *Politico*, December 11, 2020, https://www.politico.com/news/2019/12/11/azar-verma-trump-082816.

8. Yasmeen Abutaleb, Josh Dawsey, Ellen Nakashima, and Greg Miller, "The U.S. Was Beset by Denial and Dysfunction as the Coronavirus Raged," *Washington Post*, April 4, 2020, https://www.washingtonpost.com/national-security/2020/04/04/coronavirus-government-dysfunction.

9. Michael Shear, Sheri Fink, and Noah Weiland, "Inside Trump Administration, Debate Raged over What to Tell Public," *New York Times*, March 7, 2020, https://www.nytimes.com/2020/03/07/us/politics/trump-coronavirus.html.

10. Steve Eder, Henry Fountain, Michael H. Keller, Muyi Xiao, and Alexandra Stevenson, "430,000 People Have Traveled from China to U.S. Since Coronavirus Surfaced," *New York Times*, April 15, 2020, https://www.nytimes.com/2020/04/04/us/coronavirus-china-travel-restrictions.html.

11. Adam Cancryn and Sarah Owermohle, "HHS Chief Overrode FDA Officials to Ease Testing Rules," *Politico*, September 15, 2020, https://www.politico.com/news/2020/09/15/hhs-alex-azar-overrode-fda-testing-rules-415400.

12. "Remarks by President Trump, Vice President Pence, and Members of the Coronavirus Task Force in Press Conference," The White House, March 13, 2020, https://www.whitehouse.gov/briefings-statements/remarks-president-trump-vice-president-pence-members-coronavirus-task-force-press-conference-3.

13. Michael Konopasek and Rachel Skytta, "Colorado Health Officials Turn People Away from Drive-Thru COVID-19 Testing as State Struggles to Meet Demand," KDVR, Denver, March 12, 2020, https://kdvr.com/news/coronavirus/colorado-health-officials-turn-people-away-from-drive-thru-covid-19-testing-as-state-struggles-to-meet-demand.

14. Richard A. Epstein, "Why Is Health Care Special?," *University of Kansas Law Review* 40 (1992): 307–24, https://chicagounbound.uchicago.edu/cgi/viewcontent.cgi?article=2212&context=journal_articles; Richard A. Epstein, "The Kidney Crisis," Hoover Institution, October 27, 2014, https://www.hoover.org/research/kidney-crisis.

15. Isaac Chotiner, "The Contrarian Coronavirus Theory That Informed the Trump Administration," *New Yorker*, March 30, 2020, https://www.newyorker.com/news/q-and-a/the-contrarian-coronavirus-theory-that-informed-the-trump-administration.

16. Richard A. Epstein, "Coronavirus Overreaction," Hoover Institution, March 23, 2020, https://www.hoover.org/research/coronavirus-overreaction.

17. Donald J. Trump, "WE CANNOT LET THE CURE BE WORSE THAN THE PROBLEM ITSELF. AT THE END OF THE 15 DAY PERIOD, WE WILL MAKE A DECISION AS TO WHICH WAY WE WANT TO GO!," Twitter,

March 22, 2020, 11:50 p.m., https://twitter.com/realDonaldTrump/status /1241935285916782593.

18. *Munk Debates* podcast, "Be It Resolved: The Public Health Response to COVID-19 Should Focus on Protecting the Old and Letting the Young Get On with Living Normal Lives," https://munkdebates.com/podcast/us -election-%E2%80%93-pandemic-response.

19. Sarah Mervosh, Denise Lu, and Vanessa Swales, "See Which States and Cities Have Told Residents to Stay at Home," *New York Times*, last updated April 20, 2020, https://www.nytimes.com/interactive/2020/us/coronavirus-stay-at -home-order.html.

20. Kevin Breuninger, "Trump Wants 'Packed Churches' and Economy Open Again on Easter Despite the Deadly Threat of Coronavirus," CNBC, March 24, 2020, https://www.cnbc.com/2020/03/24/coronavirus-response-trump-wants-to -reopen-us-economy-by-easter.html.

21. Justin Davidson, "The Leader of the Free World Gives a Speech, and She Nails It," *New York Magazine*, https://nymag.com/intelligencer/2020/03/angela -merkel-nails-coronavirus-speech-unlike-trump.html.

22. Caitlin Oprysko and Susannah Luthi, "Trump Labels Himself 'A Wartime Politician' Combating Coronavirus," *Politico*, March 18, 2020, https://www .politico.com/news/2020/03/18/trump-administration-self-swab-coronavirus -tests-135590.

23. Elizabeth Harris, "How 'Rage' Challenged Bob Woodward," *New York Times*, September 30, 2020, https://www.nytimes.com/2020/09/30/books/bob -woodward-rage-donald-trump.html.

24. Harvey V. Fineberg, "Ten Weeks to Crush the Curve," *New England Journal of Medicine* 382, no. 17 (April 23, 2020): e37, https://doi.org/10.1056 /NEJMe2007263; National Academies of Sciences, Engineering, and Medicine, "Rapid Expert Consultation on the Possibility of Bioaerosol Spread of SARS-CoV-2 for the COVID-19 Pandemic," April 1, 2020, https://doi.org/10.17226 /25769; Elizabeth Cohen, "Experts Tell White House Coronavirus Can Spread Through Talking or Even Just Breathing," CNN, April 4, 2020, https://www .cnn.com/2020/04/02/health/aerosol-coronavirus-spread-white-house-letter /index.html; Harvey V. Fineberg, Jim Yong Kim, and Jordan Shlain, "The United States Needs a 'Smart Quarantine' to Stop the Virus Spread Within Families," *New York Times*, April 7, 2020, https://www.nytimes.com/2020/04/07/opinion /coronavirus-smart-quarantine.html.

Chapter 5: The Virus and the White House, Part II

1. Anagha Srikanth, "Who Is Coronavirus Warrior Dr. Deborah Birx?," *The Hill*, March 26, 2020, https://thehill.com/changing-america/well-being/prevention -cures/489717-who-is-coronavirus-warrior-dr-deborah-birx.

2. Nicholas Reich and Caitlin Rivers, "Scientists Want to Predict Covid-19's Long-Term Trajectory. Here's Why They Can't," *Washington Post*, September 15, 2020, https://www.washingtonpost.com/outlook/2020/09/15/scientists-want-predict-covid-19s-long-term-trajectory-heres-why-they-cant.

3. "COVID-19 Model FAQs," Institute for Health Metrics and Evaluation, March 24, 2020, http://www.healthdata.org/covid/faqs.

4. "New IHME Forecast Projects Nearly 135,000 COVID-19 Deaths in US," Institute for Health Metrics and Evaluation, May 4, 2020, http://www.healthdata.org/news-release/new-ihme-forecast-projects-nearly-135000-covid-19-deaths-us.

5. Maegan Vazquez, "Trump Estimates US Coronavirus Death Toll Will Be Lower Than Earlier Projections," CNN, April 21, 2020, https://www.cnn.com/world/live-news/coronavirus-pandemic-04-21-20-intl/h_a266b6f5fe37b3cc58cbd6c1655c0c84.

6. "Remarks by President Trump Before Marine One Departure," The White House, accessed May 5, 2020, https://www.whitehouse.gov/briefings-statements/remarks-president-trump-marine-one-departure-89.

7. "I Got COVID-19 from the White House (with Michael Shear)," *In the Bubble with Andy Slavitt*, October 28, 2020, https://podcasts.apple.com/us/podcast/i-got-covid-19-from-the-white-house-with-michael-shear/id1504128553?i=1000496327228.

8. Maggie Haberman and David E. Sanger, "Trump Says Coronavirus Cure Cannot 'Be Worse Than the Problem Itself,'" *New York Times*, March 23, 2020, https://www.nytimes.com/2020/03/23/us/politics/trump-coronavirus-restrictions.html.

9. Tyler Clifford, Jennifer Elias, and Amanda Macias, "Coronavirus Updates: Dr. Birx Outlines Phases to Reopen US Economy," CNBC, April 16, 2020, https://www.cnbc.com/2020/04/16/coronavirus-live-updates.html.

10. Robin Foster and E. J. Mundell, "Trump Says Federal Guidelines on Social Distancing Set to Expire," *U.S. News and World Report*, April 30, 2020, https://www.usnews.com/news/health-news/articles/2020–04–30/trump-says-federal-guidelines-on-social-distancing-set-to-expire.

11. Michael D. Shear et al., "Inside Trump's Failure: The Rush to Abandon Leadership Role on the Virus," *New York Times*, September 15, 2020, https://www.nytimes.com/2020/07/18/us/politics/trump-coronavirus-response-failure-leadership.html; Michael Warren, Jamie Gangel, and Elizabeth Stuart, "Jared Kushner Bragged in April That Trump Was Taking the Country 'Back from the Doctors,'" CNN, October 28, 2020, https://www.cnn.com/2020/10/28/politics/woodward-kushner-coronavirus-doctors/index.html.

Chapter 6: Trump Eats the Marshmallow

1. Rui-Heng Xu et al., "Epidemiologic Clues to SARS Origin in China," *Emerging Infectious Diseases* 10, no. 6 (June 2004): 1030–37, https://doi .org/10.3201/eid1006.030852; Kashmira Gander, "Wuhan Seafood Market Probably Wasn't Origin of Coronavirus Pandemic, Chinese Scientists Say," *Newsweek*, May 29, 2020, https://www.newsweek.com/wuhan-seafood -market-probably-wasnt-origin-coronavirus-pandemic-chinese-scientists -say-1507306.
2. Ed Yong, "How a Pandemic Might Play Out Under Trump," *The Atlantic*, December 20, 2016, https://www.theatlantic.com/science/archive/2016/12 /outbreaks-trump-disease-epidemic-ebola/511127.
3. Arnold Kling, "Stanford Marshmallow Experiment," *EconLog*, October 5, 2007, https://www.econlib.org/archives/2007/10/stanford_marshm.html.
4. "Let's Throw the Kitchen Sink at Covid-19 and Get Back to Normal by October," editorial, *Washington Post*, July 27, 2020, https://www.washingtonpost .com/opinions/what-it-would-take-to-get-back-to-normal-by-october/2020 /07/27/a8886854-d02d-11ea-8c55–61e7fa5e82ab_story.html.
5. Aaron Blake, "Trump's Disinfectant and UV Ideas Are Part of a Habit of Medical Freelancing," *Washington Post*, April 24, 2020, https://www .washingtonpost.com/politics/2020/04/24/dr-donalds-long-history-medical -freelancing.
6. Michael D. Shear et al., "Inside Trump's Failure: The Rush to Abandon Leadership Role on the Virus," *New York Times*, September 15, 2020, https://www .nytimes.com/2020/07/18/us/politics/trump-coronavirus-response-failure -leadership.html.
7. "Opening Up America Again," The White House, accessed October 13, 2020, https://www.whitehouse.gov/openingamerica.
8. Donald J. Trump, "LIBERATE MICHIGAN!," Twitter, April 17, 2020, 11:22 a.m., https://twitter.com/realDonaldTrump/status/1251169217531056130; Donald J. Trump, "LIBERATE MINNESOTA!," Twitter, April 17, 2020, 11:21 a.m., https://twitter.com/realDonaldTrump/status/1251168994066944003.
9. "Mini-Episode: American Response to COVID-19 (with David Frum)," *In the Bubble with Andy Slavitt*, May 4, 2020, https://www.lemonadamedia .com/podcast/in-the-bubble-david-frum. The quote is from the transcript of the unedited version of that episode, https://docs.google.com/document/d /1vRubB4dAy-FjhjoEn3MrTDya2iPR4NjqoOQ3c2MDQCY/edit.
10. Sen Pei, Sasikiran Kandula, and Jeffrey Shaman, "Differential Effects of Intervention Timing on COVID-19 Spread in the United States," preprint, MedRxiv, posted May 29, 2020, https://doi.org/10.1101/2020.05.15.20103655.
11. Lauren Egan, "Trump Says He Thinks Coronavirus Will 'Just Disappear' Despite Rising Cases," NBC News, July 1, 2020, https://www.nbcnews.com

/politics/white-house/trump-says-he-thinks-coronavirus-will-just-disappear
-despite-rising-n1232709.

12. Paul P. Murphy and Devan Cole, "Washington Post: WH Nixed Plan to Distribute 650 Million Face Masks Through USPS," CNN, September 18, 2020, https://
www.cnn.com/2020/09/18/politics/postal-service-face-masks-coronavirus
-trump-administration/index.html.

13. Catharine Richert, "Behind Rallies to Reopen Economy, a Minnesota Activist and His Family," MPR News, April 20, 2020, https://www.mprnews
.org/story/2020/04/20/behind-calls-to-reopen-economy-a-mn-activist-and
-his-family.

14. Isaac Stanley-Becker and Tony Romm, "Pro-Gun Activists Using Facebook
Groups to Push Anti-Quarantine Protests," *Washington Post*, April 19, 2020,
https://www.washingtonpost.com/technology/2020/04/19/pro-gun-activists
-using-facebook-groups-push-anti-quarantine-protests.

15. Brandy Zadrozny and Ben Collins, "Conservative Activist Family Behind
'Grassroots' Anti-Quarantine Facebook Events," NBC News, April 20, 2020,
https://www.nbcnews.com/tech/social-media/conservative-activist-family
-behind-grassroots-anti-quarantine-facebook-events-n1188021.

16. "What Should States Do Next? With Governor Gretchen Whitmer," *In the
Bubble with Andy Slavitt*, June 24, 2020, https://www.lemonadamedia.com
/podcast/what-should-states-do-next-with-governor-gretchen-whitmer.

17. Evan Hill, Ainara Tiefenthäler, Christiaan Triebert, Drew Jordan, Haley Willis,
and Robin Stein, "8 Minutes and 46 Seconds: How George Floyd Was Killed
in Police Custody," *New York Times*, May 31, 2020, https://www.nytimes.com
/2020/05/31/us/george-floyd-investigation.html.

18. Quint Forgey, "Trump Threatens to Unleash Gunfire on Minnesota Protesters," *Politico*, May 29, 2020, https://www.politico.com/news/2020/05/29/trump
-threatens-to-unleash-gunfire-on-minnesota-protesters-288406.

19. Will Feuer, "WHO Says There's 'No Empirical Evidence' Trump-Touted Hydroxychloroquine Helps Treat or Prevent Coronavirus," CNBC, May 27, 2020,
https://www.cnbc.com/2020/05/27/who-says-no-empirical-evidence-trump
-touted-hydroxychloroquine-helps-treat-or-prevent-coronavirus.html.

20. Tory Newmyer, "The Finance 202: Goldman Sachs Says Wearing Face
Masks Could Save the Economy," *Washington Post*, July 1, 2020, https://
www.washingtonpost.com/news/powerpost/paloma/the-finance-202/2020
/07/01/the-finance-202-goldman-sachs-says-wearing-face-masks-could-save
-the-economy/5efbc17388e0fa7b44f6b7f9; Herb Scribner, "Coronavirus:
Can Wearing a Mask Help the Economy? Yes, Kaplan Says," *Deseret News*,
July 12, 2020, https://www.deseret.com/u-s-world/2020/7/12/21319973
/coronavirus-economy-face-masks-covid-19; "Coronavirus' Business Impact:
Evolving Perspective," McKinsey, accessed October 18, 2020, https://www

.mckinsey.com/business-functions/risk/our-insights/covid-19-implications-for
-business.

21. Lauren Aratani, "How Did Face Masks Become a Political Issue in America?,"
Guardian, June 29, 2020, https://www.theguardian.com/world/2020/jun/29
/face-masks-us-politics-coronavirus.

22. Zeynep Tufekci, "How Hong Kong Did It," *The Atlantic*, May 12, 2020,
https://www.theatlantic.com/technology/archive/2020/05/how-hong-kong
-beating-coronavirus/611524.

23. Wei Lyu and George L. Wehby, "Community Use of Face Masks and
COVID-19: Evidence from a Natural Experiment of State Mandates in the
US," *Health Affairs* 39, no. 8 (June 16, 2020), https://www.healthaffairs.org
/doi/10.1377/hlthaff.2020.00818.

24. Anthony Zurcher, "Coronavirus: Who Trump Supporters Blame for Virus
'Hysteria,'" BBC News, March 11, 2020, https://www.bbc.com/news/world
-us-canada-51840227.

25. Julianne Holt-Lunstad, "The Double Pandemic of Social Isolation and
COVID-19: Cross-Sector Policy Must Address Both," Health Affairs Blog,
June 22, 2020, https://www.healthaffairs.org/do/10.1377/hblog20200609
.53823.

26. Zurcher, "Coronavirus."

27. "'The Death Threats Started Last Month': Public Health Officials Targeted by
Some Frustrated Americans," *Kaiser Health News*, June 23, 2020, https://khn
.org/morning-breakout/the-death-threats-started-last-month-public-health
-officials-targeted-by-some-frustrated-americans.

28. Christina Carrega, Veronica Stracqualursi, and Josh Campbell, "Gretchen
Whitmer: 13 Charged in Plot to Kidnap Michigan Governor," CNN, October 10, 2020, https://www.cnn.com/2020/10/08/politics/fbi-plot-michigan
-governor-gretchen-whitmer/index.html.

29. "Toolkit: How to Talk to Each Other About Wearing Masks," *In the Bubble
with Andy Slavitt*, June 29, 2020, https://www.lemonadamedia.com/podcast
/toolkit-how-to-talk-to-each-other-about-masks.

Chapter 7: No One Left in Charge but the Virus

1. Steven Brill, "Obama's Trauma Team," *Time*, February 27, 2014, https://time
.com/10228/obamas-trauma-team.

2. "Tracking Our COVID-19 Response," Covid Exit Strategy, accessed October
13, 2020, https://www.covidexitstrategy.org.

3. Dasia Moore and Kay Lazar, "In Pandemic Recovery, New York Has Had More
Success than Mass. What Explains the Gap?," *Boston Globe*, August 16, 2020,
https://www.bostonglobe.com/2020/08/16/nation/beating-back-covid-19-new
-york-emerges-leader.

4. CNN Transcripts, *Cuomo Prime Time*, CNN, May 7, 2020, http://transcripts .cnn.com/TRANSCRIPTS/2005/07/CPT.01.html.

5. Andy Slavitt, "Relaxing All Social Distancing Behaviors Now Is a Huge Mistake," Medium Coronavirus Blog, May 2, 2020, https://coronavirus.medium .com/relaxing-all-social-distancing-behaviors-now-is-a-huge-mistake -c03674423888. Lightly edited for its inclusion in this book.

6. Michael D. Shear, Noah Weiland, Eric Lipton, Maggie Haberman, and David E. Sanger, "Inside Trump's Failure: The Rush to Abandon Leadership Role on the Virus," *New York Times*, September 15, 2020, https://www.nytimes.com /2020/07/18/us/politics/trump-coronavirus-response-failure-leadership.html.

7. MSNBC, "President Trump on Coronavirus Testing: 'I Said to My People, Slow the Testing Down, Please,'" Twitter, June 20, 2020, 9:03 p.m., https:// twitter.com/MSNBC/status/1274508151086370816.

8. Andy Slavitt, "COVID Update June 18: Even as surges start to hit the South and West, all states must prepare for what's next," Twitter, June 18, 2020, 9:25 p.m., https://twitter.com/ASlavitt/status/1273789055705264129.

9. "The Best Thing Everyday Americans Can Do to Fight Coronavirus? #Stay-Home, Save Lives," *USA Today*, March 15, 2020, https://www.usatoday.com /story/opinion/2020/03/15/coronavirus-stay-home-hel-america-save-lives -column/5054241002.

10. "Our Data," COVID Tracking Project, accessed September 27, 2020, https:// covidtracking.com/data; "COVIDView, Key Updates for Week 22," Centers for Disease Control and Prevention, June 5, 2020, https://www.cdc.gov /coronavirus/2019-ncov/covid-data/covidview/past-reports/06052020.html.

11. Julie Bosman and Mitch Smith, "Coronavirus Cases Spike Across Sun Belt as Economy Lurches into Motion," *New York Times*, June 18, 2020, https:// www.nytimes.com/2020/06/14/us/coronavirus-united-states.html.

12. Langston Taylor, "Florida Coronavirus Data Manager Was Told to Remove Data Before Reassignment, Emails Show," *Tampa Bay Times*, May 19, 2020, https://www.tampabay.com/news/health/2020/05/19/florida-health-department-officials-told-manager-to-delete-coronavirus-data-before -reassigning-her-emails-show. She later went on to release the data herself: Laurel Wamsley, "Fired Florida Data Scientist Launches a Coronavirus Dashboard of Her Own," NPR, June 14, 2020, https://www.npr.org/2020/06/14 /876584284/fired-florida-data-scientist-launches-a-coronavirus-dashboard -of-her-own.

13. "Trends in U.S. Income and Wealth Inequality," Pew Research Center, Social and Demographic Trends Project, January 9, 2020, https://www .pewsocialtrends.org/2020/01/09/trends-in-income-and-wealth-inequality; Cecelia Smith-Schoenwalder, "Florida Suspends Alcohol Consumption at Bars Amid Coronavirus Surge," *U.S. News and World Report*, June 26, 2020,

https://www.usnews.com/news/health-news/articles/2020–06–26/florida
-suspends-alcohol-consumption-at-bars-amid-coronavirus-surge; Arek Sarkis-
sian, "Florida to Reopen Bars, Pack Restaurants After DeSantis Claims
Covid-19 Under Control," *Politico*, September 10, 2020, https://www.politico
.com/states/florida/story/2020/09/10/desantis-will-let-florida-restaurants
-pack-dining-rooms-soon-1316481.

14. House Committee on Appropriations, "H.R.6800—The Heroes Act," Library of
Congress, May 12, 2020, https://www.congress.gov/bill/116th-congress/house
-bill/6800.

15. Alexa Block, "Looking Back at the Timeline of Coronavirus in Arizona," 12
News (Phoenix), September 28, 2020, https://www.12news.com/article/news
/local/arizona/timeline-of-coronavirus-in-arizona/75–69c216df-6773–4b25
-a34d-5a397d049196.

16. Amit Syal, "Congressman Ruben Gallego and Two Health Experts Hold Press
Conference for Spike in COVID-19 Cases," *Daily Wildcat*, June 15, 2020, https://
www.wildcat.arizona.edu/article/2020/06/sc-congressman-press-conference.

17. Laurie Roberts, "Doug Ducey Admits Arizona Is in Trouble on COVID-19
but Does Nothing," *AZCentral*, June 25, 2020, https://www.azcentral.com
/story/opinion/op-ed/laurieroberts/2020/06/25/doug-ducey-admits-arizona
-trouble-coronavirus-does-nothing/3261731001.

18. Jeff Popovich, "Arizona to Close Bars, Gyms, Theaters Again; Delay Start of
School," *AZFamily*, June 29, 2020, https://www.azfamily.com/news/continuing
_coverage/coronavirus_coverage/arizona-to-close-bars-gyms-theaters-again
-delay-start-of-school/article_663e8f2e-ba4c-11ea-a9b4-b7d21d07fe73.html;
"Our Data."

19. Stephen Groves, "Noem Says South Dakota Is Doing 'Good' as Virus Surges,"
Associated Press, October 22, 2020, https://apnews.com/article/virus-outbreak
-health-south-dakota-f967a1a56b798f43ae0d2be971b27b39.

20. Molly Gamble, "States Ranked by COVID-19 Test Positivity Rates: Nov.
5," *Becker's Hospital Review*, accessed November 6, 2020, https://www
.beckershospitalreview.com/public-health/states-ranked-by-covid-19-test
-positivity-rates-july-14.html.

21. "Birx Warns That U.S. Epidemic Is in a 'New Phase,'" *New York Times*, August 4, 2020, https://www.nytimes.com/2020/08/02/world/coronavirus-covid
-19.html.

22. Elizabeth Thomas, "The New Doctor in Trump's Pandemic Response Briefings:
Scott Atlas Agrees with Him on Masks, Opening Schools," ABC News, August
14, 2020, https://abcnews.go.com/Politics/doctor-trumps-pandemic-response
-briefings-scott-atlas-agrees/story?id=72376728.

23. Andy Slavitt, "We need to increase test capacity more. University labs should
get rapid CLIA certification. Pooling samples and large scale saliva tests will

help but are still some time off," Twitter, July 3, 2020, 2:00 p.m., https://twitter.com/aslavitt/status/1279112764280225792.

24. COVID Tracking Project, "Our Data."

25. Jason Beaubien, "Americans Are Dying in the Pandemic at Rates Far Higher Than in Other Countries," NPR, October 10, 2020, https://www.npr.org/sections/health-shots/2020/10/13/923253681/americans-are-dying-in-the-pandemic-at-rates-far-higher-than-in-other-countries.

Chapter 8: The Room Service Pandemic

1. TPNS, "Dr. King's Last Christmas Sermon," MLK Global, December 23, 2017, https://mlkglobal.org/2017/12/23/dr-kings-last-christmas-sermon.

2. Joe Hansen, "The Moral Test of Government," *HuffPost*, September 3, 2012, https://www.huffpost.com/entry/the-moral-test-of-governm_b_1847379.

3. "The History and Evolution of CHIP and the Medicare Program," HealthPayerIntelligence, December 30, 2015, https://healthpayerintelligence.com/news/the-history-and-evolution-of-chip-and-the-medicare-program.

4. "Family Separations at US Border Plagued by Problems, Watchdog Finds," *Guardian*, March 6, 2020, http://www.theguardian.com/us-news/2020/mar/06/trump-border-separations-children-mexico-watchdog; Katie Keith, "HHS Strips Gender Identity, Sex Stereotyping, Language Access Protections from ACA Anti-Discrimination Rule," Health Affairs Blog, June 13, 2020, https://www.healthaffairs.org/do/10.1377/hblog20200613.671888/full; Tucker Higgins, "Supreme Court Allows Trump's 'Public Charge' Immigration Rule," CNBC, January 27, 2020, https://www.cnbc.com/2020/01/27/supreme-court-allows-trumps-public-charge-immigration-rule.html; Lola Fadulu, "Medicaid Work Requirements: Do They Actually Help?," *The Atlantic*, April 12, 2019, https://www.theatlantic.com/health/archive/2019/04/medicaid-work-requirements-seema-verma-cms/587026.

5. Terri Lobdell, "Office for Civil Rights: Why Is It There and What Does It Do?," Palo Alto Online, June 14, 2013, https://www.paloaltoonline.com/news/2013/06/14/office-for-civil-rights-why-is-it-there-and-what-does-it-do; "Conscience Protections for Health Care Providers," Office for Civil Rights, Department of Health and Human Services, October 14, 2010, https://www.hhs.gov/conscience/conscience-protections/index.html.

6. Scott Neuman, "COVID-19 Death Rate for Black Americans Twice That for Whites, New Report Says," NPR, August 13, 2020, https://www.npr.org/sections/coronavirus-live-updates/2020/08/13/902261618/covid-19-death-rate-for-black-americans-twice-that-for-whites-new-report-says; "Johns Hopkins Report," State of Black Empowerment, accessed October 14, 2020, https://soba.iamempowered.com/johns-hopkins-report.

7. "About Dan Patrick Lieutenant Governor," Lieutenant Governor Dan Patrick, accessed October 14, 2020, https://ltgweb/about.

8. Richard Whittaker, "Dan Patrick Excoriated over Orlando Shooting Tweet: Lite Guv Blames Twitter Debacle on Timing, Not Bigotry," *Austin Chronicle*, June 12, 2016, https://www.austinchronicle.com/daily/news/2016-06-12/dan-patrick-excoriated-over-orlando-shooting-tweet.

9. Sanford Nowlin, "Lt. Gov. Dan Patrick Uses Anti-Gay Slur to Describe Beto O'Rourke During Fox News Interview," *San Antonio Current*, April 30, 2019, https://www.sacurrent.com/the-daily/archives/2019/04/30/ltgov-dan-patrick-uses-anti-gay-slur-to-describe-beto-orourke-during-fox-news-interview.

10. Alex Samuels, "Dan Patrick Says Opening Economy Is More Important Than Saving Lives," *Texas Tribune*, April 21, 2020, https://www.texastribune.org/2020/04/21/texas-dan-patrick-economy-coronavirus.

11. "Who Are We Asking to Die? With Beto O'Rourke," *In the Bubble with Andy Slavitt*, May 13, 2020, https://www.lemonadamedia.com/podcast/in-the-bubble-beto-orourke.

12. Timothy Williams and Danielle Ivory, "Coronavirus Behind Bars: Cook County Jail Is Top U.S. Hot Spot," *New York Times*, April 8, 2020, https://www.nytimes.com/2020/04/08/us/coronavirus-cook-county-jail-chicago.html; "COVID-19 Cases at CCDOC," Cook County Sheriff's Office, accessed October 14, 2020, https://www.cookcountysheriff.org/covid-19-cases-at-ccdoc.

13. Prison Policy Initiative, "How Many People Are Locked Up in the United States?," accessed October 23, 2020, https://www.prisonpolicy.org/graphs/pie2020.html.

14. Harmeet Kaur and Stella Chan, "San Quentin Coronavirus Outbreak: At Least 15 Inmates Have Died of Apparent Complications from Covid-19," CNN, July 23, 2020, https://www.cnn.com/2020/07/23/us/california-san-quentin-coronavirus-inmates-trnd/index.html.

15. David Waldstein, "C.D.C. Stresses Need for Coronavirus Testing at Homeless Shelters," *New York Times*, April 23, 2020, https://www.nytimes.com/2020/04/23/health/coronavirus-testing-homeless-shelters.html.

16. "South Dakota Meatpacking Plant Becomes Nation's Top Coronavirus Hotspot as Governor Shuns Stay-at-Home Order," CBS News, April 15, 2020, https://www.cbsnews.com/news/south-dakota-coronavirus-cases-smithfield-foods-plant-governor-kristi-noem-shuns-stay-at-home-order-2020-04-15.

17. Hollie Silverman, Konstantin Toropin, Sara Sidner, and Leslie Perrot, "Navajo Nation Surpasses New York State for Highest Covid-19 Infection Rate in the US," CNN, May 18, 2020, https://www.cnn.com/2020/05/18/us/navajo-nation

-infection-rate-trnd/index.html; "In Numbers: COVID-19 Across the Navajo Nation," *Navajo Times*, accessed October 14, 2020, https://navajotimes.com/coronavirus-updates/covid-19-across-the-navajo-nation.

18. Laurel Morales, "Navajo Nation Sees High Rate of COVID-19 and Contact Tracing Is a Challenge," NPR, April 24, 2020, https://www.npr.org/2020/04/24/842945050/navajo-nation-sees-high-rate-of-covid-19-and-contact-tracing-is-a-challenge.

19. Katy Read, "Morgan Yesnes, Who Focused on Living Every Day Despite Terminal Illnesses, Dies at 24," *Star Tribune*, May 17, 2020, https://www.startribune.com/morgan-yesnes-who-focused-on-living-every-day-despite-terminal-illnesses-dies-at-24/570536392.

20. "How a Small Wedding in Maine Became a Deadly COVID-19 Superspreader," *Healthline*, September 21, 2020, https://www.healthline.com/health-news/how-a-small-wedding-in-maine-became-a-deadly-covid-19-superspreader; Associated Press, "Maine 'Superspreader' Wedding Linked to 170 Covid Cases and Seven Deaths," *Guardian*, September 17, 2020, https://www.theguardian.com/us-news/2020/sep/17/maine-wedding-superspreader-event.

21. Sarah Holder, "Why Are Americans So Uneasy About Contact Tracing?," Bloomberg, August 12, 2020, https://www.bloomberg.com/news/articles/2020–08–12/why-are-americans-so-uneasy-about-contact-tracing.

22. Associated Press, "MN COVID-19 Testing Options Abound, but with Waits," *Independent* (Marshall, MN), September 8, 2020, https://www.marshallindependent.com/news/minnesota-news-apwire/2020/09/mn-covid-19-testing-options-abound-but-with-waits; Jeremy Olson, "COVID-19 Tally Inflated by Lab's Delay, Large Events," *Star Tribune*, August 28, 2020, https://m.startribune.com/delayed-lab-reporting-bumps-up-minnesota-virus-numbers/572239492.

23. Benjamin Siegel, Mark Abdelmalek, and Jay Bhatt, "Coronavirus Contact Tracers' Nemeses: People Who Don't Answer Their Phones," ABC News, May 15, 2020, https://abcnews.go.com/Health/coronavirus-contact-tracers-nemeses-people-answer-phones/story?id=70693586.

24. "US States with the Most Essential Workers," United Way of the National Capital Area, accessed October 14, 2020, https://unitedwaynca.org/stories/us-states-essential-workers.

25. Paul John Scott, "'We're Going to See Changing COVID-19 Information,' Minnesota Lawmakers Are Told," *West Central Tribune*, July 8, 2020, https://www.wctrib.com/newsmd/coronavirus/6566377-Were-going-to-see-changing-COVID-19-information-Minnesota-lawmakers-are-told.

26. "The Economic Tracker," accessed November 9, 2020, https://tracktherecovery.org.

27. Andy Slavitt, "In the future, definitions in @Dictionarycom are going to need to include what 'essential worker' came to mean during the COVID crisis," Twitter, July 7, 2020, 7:15 p.m., https://twitter.com/ASlavitt/status /1280641670250467336. Lightly edited for use here.

28. Sanjay Bhandari, Aprill Z. Dawson, Rebekah J. Walker, and Leonard E. Egede, "Elderly African Americans: The Vulnerable of the Vulnerable in the COVID-19 Era," *Aging Medicine*, October 22, 2020, https://onlinelibrary.wiley.com/doi /full/10.1002/agm2.12131.

29. Higgins, "Supreme Court Allows Trump's 'Public Charge' Immigration Rule."

30. "Labor Force Characteristics by Race and Ethnicity, 2018," Report 1082, U.S. Bureau of Labor Statistics, October 2019, https://www.bls.gov/opub/reports /race-and-ethnicity/2018/home.htm.

31. "COVID-19 Deaths Analyzed by Race and Ethnicity," APM Research Lab, accessed October 14, 2020, https://www.apmresearchlab.org/covid/deaths -by-race; Tiffany N. Ford, Sarah Reber, and Richard V. Reeves, "Race Gaps in COVID-19 Deaths Are Even Bigger Than They Appear," Brookings Institution, June 16, 2020, https://www.brookings.edu/blog/up-front/2020/06/16 /race-gaps-in-covid-19-deaths-are-even-bigger-than-they-appear.

32. Greg Asbed, "What Happens If America's 2.5 Million Farmworkers Get Sick?," *New York Times*, April 3, 2020, https://www.nytimes.com/2020/04/03/opinion /coronavirus-farm-workers.html.

33. "California Coronavirus Cases: Tracking the Outbreak," *Los Angeles Times*, accessed October 14, 2020, https://www.latimes.com/projects/california -coronavirus-cases-tracking-outbreak.

34. "Racial and Ethnic Disparities in Diabetes Prevalence, Self-Management, and Health Outcomes Among Medicare Beneficiaries," March 2017, https://www.cms.gov/About-CMS/Agency-Information/OMH/research -and-data/information-products/data-highlights/disparities-in-diabetes -prevalence.

35. "The Root Causes of Health Inequity," chapter 3 in *Communities in Action: Pathways to Health Equity* (Washington, DC: National Academies Press, 2017), https://www.ncbi.nlm.nih.gov/books/NBK425845.

36. Janice A. Sabin, "How We Fail Black Patients in Pain," AAMC, January 6, 2020, https://www.aamc.org/news-insights/how-we-fail-black-patients-pain.

37. Mary M. Chapman, "As Detroit Suffers, Black Workers Hurt," *New York Times*, December 30, 2008, https://www.nytimes.com/2008/12/30/business /30detroit.html.

38. Jordan Rau, "Trump Administration Eases Nursing Home Fines in Victory for Industry," *New York Times*, December 24, 2017, https://www.nytimes.com /2017/12/24/business/trump-administration-nursing-home-penalties.html.

39. Elaine K. Howley, "Nursing Home Facts and Statistics," *U.S. News and World Report*, accessed October 14, 2020, https://health.usnews.com/health-news/best-nursing-homes/articles/nursing-home-facts-and-statistics.

40. Ricardo Alonso-Zaldivar, "Report: Much Needs Doing to Shield Nursing Homes from Virus," Associated Press, September 17, 2020, https://apnews.com/article/virus-outbreak-michael-pence-archive-nursing-homes-donald-trump-dc63932d7aca280feda372459ebd608e.

41. "Kansas Prisoners Riot Transcript: 4/10/20," *The Rachel Maddow Show*, MSNBC, April 10, 2020, https://www.msnbc.com/transcripts/rachel-maddow-show/2020-04-10-msna1347831.

42. Charlotta Stern and Daniel B. Klein, "Stockholm City's Elderly Care and Covid19: Interview with Barbro Karlsson," *Society* 57 (July 19, 2020): 434–45, https://doi.org/10.1007/s12115-020-00508-0; Carl-Johann Karlsson, "Sweden's Failure to Protect Its Elderly Population from Coronavirus Started Long Before the Pandemic," *Foreign Policy*, June 23, 2020, https://foreignpolicy.com/2020/06/23/sweden-coronavirus-failure-anders-tegnell-started-long-before-the-pandemic.

43. "Size and Demographics of Aging Populations," chapter 2 in Institute of Medicine, *Providing Healthy and Safe Foods as We Age: Workshop Summary* (Washington, DC: National Academies Press, 2010), https://www.ncbi.nlm.nih.gov/books/NBK51841.

44. Emma Reynolds, "Elderly People and Coronavirus: It's the Worst Disaster of the Pandemic. But WHO Chief Says Our Lack of Concern Shows 'Moral Bankruptcy,'" CNN, September 4, 2020, https://www.cnn.com/2020/09/04/health/elderly-care-coronavirus-who-tedros-intl/index.html.

45. Long H. Nguyen et al., "Risk of COVID-19 Among Front-Line Health-Care Workers and the General Community: A Prospective Cohort Study," *Lancet Public Health* 5 (2020): e475–83, https://www.thelancet.com/journals/lanpub/article/PIIS2468-2667(20)30164-X/fulltext#seccestitle140.

46. "Lost on the Frontline: US Healthcare Workers Who Died Fighting Covid-19," *Guardian*, accessed October 14, 2020, https://www.theguardian.com/us-news/ng-interactive/2020/aug/11/lost-on-the-frontline-covid-19-coronavirus-us-healthcare-workers-deaths-database.

Chapter 9: The Folly of the Free Market Pandemic

1. Saloni Sardana, "US Billionaires' Wealth Grew by $845 Billion During the First Six Months of the Pandemic," *Business Insider*, September 17, 2020, https://www.businessinsider.com/us-billionaires-wealth-net-worth-pandemic-covid-billion-2020-9.

2. Mary Chapin Carpenter, "The Bug," accessed November 8, 2020, https://genius.com/Mary-chapin-carpenter-the-bug-lyrics.

3. "Statistics: The Kidney Project," University of California–San Francisco, accessed November 9, 2020, https://pharm.ucsf.edu/kidney/need/statistics.

4. Edward Salsberg and Robert Martiniano, "Health Care Jobs Projected to Continue to Grow Far Faster Than Jobs in the General Economy," Health Affairs Blog, May 9, 2018, https://www.healthaffairs.org/do/10.1377/hblog20180502.984593/full.

5. Cheryl Barton, "Annual Revenue of Top 10 Big Pharma Companies," *Pharma Letter*, March 3, 2020, https://www.thepharmaletter.com/article/annual-revenue-of-top-10-big-pharma-companies; Paige Minemyer, "Health Insurers' Profits Topped $35B Last Year. Medicare Advantage Is the Common Thread," *Fierce Healthcare*, February 24, 2020, https://www.fiercehealthcare..com/payer/big-name-payers-earned-35-7-billion-2019-here-s-one-common-thread-their-reports; "50 Top-Grossing For-Profit Hospitals," *Becker's Hospital Review*, June 27, 2014, https://www.beckershospitalreview.com/lists/50-top-grossing-for-profit-hospitals-2014.html.

6. "NHE Fact Sheet," Centers for Medicaid and Medicare Services, accessed February 23, 2020, https://www.cms.gov/research-statistics-data-and-systems/statistics-trends-and-reports/nationalhealthexpenddata/nhe-fact-sheet.

7. Megan Leonhardt, "Americans Now Spend Twice as Much on Health Care as They Did in the 1980s," CNBC, October 9, 2019, https://www.cnbc.com/2019/10/09/americans-spend-twice-as-much-on-health-care-today-as-in-the-1980s.html.

8. Emily Gee and Topher Spiro, "Excess Administrative Costs Burden the U.S. Health Care System," Center for American Progress, April 8, 2019, https://www.americanprogress.org/issues/healthcare/reports/2019/04/08/468302/excess-administrative-costs-burden-u-s-health-care-system.

9. Jan Berger et al., "How Drug Life-Cycle Management Patent Strategies May Impact Formulary Management," *American Journal of Managed Care* 22, no. 16 (2017), https://www.ajmc.com/view/a636-article.

10. Aimee Picchi, "Drug Prices in 2019 Are Surging, with Hikes at 5 Times Inflation," CBS News, July 1, 2019, https://www.cbsnews.com/news/drug-prices-in-2019-are-surging-with-hikes-at-5-times-inflation; Curtis E. Haas, "Drug Price Increases: Here We Go Again?," *Pharmacy Times*, March 19, 2019, https://www.pharmacytimes.com/publications/health-system-edition/2019/march2019/drug-price-increases-here-we-go-again.

11. Peter Loftus, "Drugmakers, Worried About Losing Pricing Power, Are Lobbying Hard," *Wall Street Journal*, September 24, 2019, https://www.wsj.com/articles/drugmakers-worried-about-losing-pricing-power-are-lobbying-hard-11569317406.

12. Laura Entis, "Why Does Medicine Cost So Much? Here's How Drug Prices Are Set," *Time*, April 9, 2019, https://time.com/5564547/drug-prices-medicine;

Emily Miller, "US Drug Prices vs the World," *Drugwatch*, last updated July 27, 2020, https://www.drugwatch.com/featured/us-drug-prices-higher-vs-world.

13. American Hospital Association, "Statement of the American Hospital Association Submitted to the Committee on Finance of the United States Senate on Bipartisan Tax Reform," April 15, 2015, https://www.aha.org/system/files /advocacy-issues/testimony/2015/150415-statement-taxreform.pdf.

14. Mustaqeem Siddiqui and S. Vincent Rajkumar, "The High Cost of Cancer Drugs and What We Can Do About It," *Mayo Clinic Proceedings* 87, no. 10 (October 2012): 935–43, https://doi.org/10.1016/j.mayocp.2012.07.007; J. D. McCue, C. Hansen, and P. Gal, "Hospital Charges for Antibiotics," *Reviews of Infectious Diseases* 7, no. 5 (October 1985): 643–45, https://doi.org/10.1093 /clinids/7.5.643.

15. "Global Pharmaceutical Industry—Statistics & Facts," Statista, accessed November 9, 2020, https://www.statista.com/topics/1764/global-pharmaceutical -industry.

16. Statista, "Global Pharmaceutical Industry—Statistics & Facts."

17. Beth Mole, "Big Pharma Shells Out $20B Each Year to Schmooze Docs, $6B on Drug Ads," *Ars Technica*, January 11, 2019, https://arstechnica.com /science/2019/01/healthcare-industry-spends-30b-on-marketing-most-of-it -goes-to-doctors.

18. Jeff Lagasse, "About 1 in 5 Hospitals Mark Up Drug Prices at Least 700 Percent, Study Finds," *Healthcare Finance*, September 5, 2018, https://www .healthcarefinancenews.com/news/about-1-5-hospitals-mark-drug-prices -least-700-percent-study-finds; Bob Herman, "Hospitals Are Making a Lot of Money on Outpatient Drugs," *Axios*, February 15, 2019, https://www .axios.com/hospital-charges-outpatient-drug-prices-markups-b0931c02 -a254-4876-825f-4b53b38614a3.html.

19. Jake Frankenfield, "Which Industry Spends the Most on Lobbying?," *Investopedia*, last updated May 7, 2020, https://www.investopedia.com/investing /which-industry-spends-most-lobbying-antm-so.

20. Morgan Haefner, "No More 'Heads in Beds': Outpatient Visits Outpace Inpatient, Deloitte Finds," *Becker's Hospital Review*, February 26, 2020, https:// www.beckershospitalreview.com/finance/no-more-heads-in-beds-outpatient -visits-outpace-inpatient-deloitte-finds.html.

21. Arthur H. Gale, "Bigger But Not Better: Hospital Mergers Increase Costs and Do Not Improve Quality," *Missouri Medicine* 112, no. 1 (2015): 4–5.

22. Michael A. Morrisey, Gerald J. Wedig, and Mahmud Hassan, "Do Nonprofit Hospitals Pay Their Way?," *Health Affairs* 15, no. 4 (January 1, 1996): 132–44, https://doi.org/10.1377/hlthaff.15.4.132.

23. Laura Snyder and Robin Rudowitz, "Medicaid Financing: How Does It Work and What Are the Implications?," KFF, May 20, 2015, https://www.kff.org

/medicaid/issue-brief/medicaid-financing-how-does-it-work-and-what-are-the
-implications; Jack Hadley and John Holahan, "How Much Medical Care Do
the Uninsured Use, and Who Pays for It?," *Health Affairs* 22, suppl. 1 (2003),
https://www.healthaffairs.org/doi/full/10.1377/hlthaff.W3.66; "Uncompen-
sated Health Care Costs in the United States," DECO Recovery Management,
July 29, 2019, https://www.decorm.com/uncompensated-health-care-costs-in
-the-united-states; Steven W. Kennedy Jr. and Gregory I. Sawchyn, "Financing
Options for Large Hospitals and Multi-Hospital Systems," *Becker's Hospital
Review*, December 7, 2010, https://www.beckershospitalreview.com/hospital
-management-administration/financing-options-for-large-hospitals-and-multi
-hospital-systems.html.

24. Kate Zernike, "The Hidden Subsidy That Helps Pay for Health Insurance,"
New York Times, July 7, 2017, https://www.nytimes.com/2017/07/07/health
/health-insurance-tax-deduction.html.

25. "Rate Review & the 80/20 Rule," HealthCare.gov, accessed October 14, 2020,
https://www.healthcare.gov/health-care-law-protections/rate-review; Blake
Morgan, "The Top 5 Industries Most Hated by Customers," *Forbes*, October
16, 2018, https://www.forbes.com/sites/blakemorgan/2018/10/16/top-5-most
-hated-industries-by-customers.

26. Matthew Fox, "These 3 Stocks Have Surged More Than 1,000 Percent Since
the COVID-19 Pandemic Low (OSTK, W, NVAX)," *Business Insider*, August 5,
2020, https://www.businessinsider.com/stocks-price-massive-gains-coronavirus
-covid19-low-overstock-wayfair-novavax-2020-8.

27. Alex Spanko, "AHCA's Parkinson: Nursing Homes Must 'Look in the Mirror'
to Improve Care, Infection Control Post-COVID," *Skilled Nursing News*, October 6, 2020, https://skillednursingnews.com/2020/10/ahcas-parkinson-nursing
-homes-must-look-in-the-mirror-to-improve-care-infection-control-post-covid.

28. "The Governor with the Secret Formula on COVID, with Governor Andy
Beshear," *In the Bubble with Andy Slavitt*, accessed October 14, 2020, https://
www.lemonadamedia.com/podcast/the-governor-with-the-secret-formula-on
-covid-with-governor-andy-beshear.

29. Ryan Gabrielson et al., "A Closer Look at Federal COVID Contractors Re-
veals Inexperience, Fraud Accusations and a Weapons Dealer Operating out
of Someone's House," *ProPublica*, May 27, 2020, https://www.propublica
.org/article/a-closer-look-at-federal-covid-contractors-reveals-inexperience
-fraud-accusations-and-a-weapons-dealer-operating-out-of-someones
-house.

30. "Government Cancels $55.5M Deal with Company That Had No History of
Selling Masks," *Kaiser Health News*, May 13, 2020, https://khn.org/morning
-breakout/government-cancels-55-5m-deal-with-company-that-had-no
-history-of-selling-masks.

31. "Putting People First During the Coronavirus Outbreak," press release, 3M, April 1, 2020, https://news.3m.com/English/3m-stories/3m-details/2020/Putting -people-first-during-the-coronavirus-outbreak/default.aspx.

32. Jack Nicas, "It's Bedlam in the Mask Market, as Profiteers Out-Hustle Good Samaritans," *New York Times,* April 3, 2020, https://www.nytimes.com/2020 /04/03/technology/coronavirus-masks-shortage.html.

33. Andy Slavitt, "NOW: Email, text, or call @3M and ask them how many of their masks are going to US medical community or other countries with shortages vs others? We can't needlessly lose health care workers. They must make this public. And then change," Twitter, March 29, 2020, 10:52 p.m., https://twitter .com/aslavitt/status/1244457425752776704.

34. David DiSalvo, "I Spent a Day in the Coronavirus-Driven Feeding Frenzy of N95 Mask Sellers and Buyers and This Is What I Learned," *Forbes*, March 30, 2020, https://www.forbes.com/sites/daviddisalvo/2020/03/30/i-spent-a-day-in -the-coronavirus-driven-feeding-frenzy-of-n95-mask-sellers-and-buyers-and -this-is-what-i-learned/#24531b9256d4.

35. Natasha Bertrand, Gabby Orr, Daniel Lippman, and Nahal Toosi, "Pence Task Force Freezes Coronavirus Aid amid Backlash," *Politico*, March 31, 2020, https://www.politico.com/news/2020/03/31/pence-task-force-coronavirus -aid-157806.

36. Juliet Eilperin et al., "U.S. Sent Millions of Face Masks to China Early This Year, Ignoring Pandemic Warning Signs," *Washington Post*, April 18, 2020, https://www.washingtonpost.com/health/us-sent-millions-of-face-masks -to-china-early-this-year-ignoring-pandemic-warning-signs/2020/04/18 /aaccf54a-7ff5-11ea-8013-1b6da0e4a2b7_story.html.

37. E. Tammy Kim, "How South Korea Solved Its Face Mask Shortage," *New York Times*, April 1, 2020, https://www.nytimes.com/2020/04/01/opinion/covid -face-mask-shortage.html.

38. Donald J. Trump, "We hit 3M hard today after seeing what they were doing with their Masks. 'P Act' all the way. Big surprise to many in government as to what they were doing—will have a big price to pay!," Twitter, April 2, 2020, 8:52 p.m., https://twitter.com/realDonaldTrump/status/1245876816922972162; Gavin Bade, "Trump Expands DPA, amid Mounting Pressure," *Politico*, April 2, 2020, https://www.politico.com/news/2020/04/02/trump-expands-dpa-order -162128.

39. Rachel Sandler, "Trump Ends Feud with Mask Maker 3M, Announces Deal for 55 Million U.S. Masks per Month," *Forbes*, April 6, 2020, https://www.forbes .com/sites/rachelsandler/2020/04/06/trump-ends-feud-with-mask-maker-3m -announces-deal-for-55-million-us-masks-per-month/#5dc4ed661209; Kevin Breuninger, "Trump and 3M Strike Deal to Bring 166.5 Million Masks to US in Three Months to Help Coronavirus Response," CNBC, April 6, 2020, https://

www.cnbc.com/2020/04/06/coronavirus-trump-and-3m-strike-deal-to-bring
-55point5-million-masks-a-month-to-us.html; "U.S. Government Awards $126
Million Face Masks Contract to 3M," Reuters, May 6, 2020, https://www
.reuters.com/article/us-health-coronavirus-3m-idUSKBN22I2QG.

40. "South Korea Coronavirus: 24,889 Cases and 438 Deaths," Worldometer, accessed October 14, 2020, https://www.worldometers.info/coronavirus/country
/south-korea.

41. David Morgan and Richard Cowan, "U.S. House Passes $8.3 Billion Bill to Battle
Coronavirus; Senate Vote Due Thursday," Reuters, March 5, 2020, https://www
.reuters.com/article/us-health-coronavirus-usa-congress-idUSKBN20R2V6;
Ryan Grim and Aida Chávez, "How the Senate Paved the Way for Coronavirus Profiteering," The Intercept, March 2, 2020, https://theintercept.com/2020
/03/02/coronavirus-vaccine-price-gouging-senate; Sydney Lupkin, "Prices for
COVID-19 Vaccines Are Starting to Come into Focus," NPR, August 6, 2020,
https://www.npr.org/sections/health-shots/2020/08/06/899869278/prices-for
-covid-19-vaccines-are-starting-to-come-into-focus.

42. Ed Silverman, "Azar Has a 'Tin Ear' When It Comes to Pricing a Potential
Coronavirus Vaccine," Stat, February 27, 2020, https://www.statnews.com
/2020/02/27/azar-coronavirus-affordable-trump.

43. "Fidelity, Flagship Alter Investments in Coronavirus Vaccine Maker Moderna," Boston Business Journal, August 25, 2020, https://www.bizjournals
.com/boston/news/2020/08/25/as-flagship-shrinks-moderna-holdings-fidelity
-bul.html.

44. Stephen Gandel, "Moderna Executives Hiked Their Stock Sales After Announcing Positive Vaccine Trial," CBS News, July 21, 2020, https://www.cbsnews
.com/news/moderna-executives-increased-stock-sales-after-coronavirus
-vaccine-trial-data.

45. Peter Loftus, "Moderna Vows to Not Enforce Covid-19 Vaccine Patents During
Pandemic," Wall Street Journal, October 8, 2020, https://www.wsj.com/articles
/moderna-vows-to-not-enforce-covid-19-vaccine-patents-during-pandemic
-11602154805.

46. Greg Slabodkin, "CMS Doubles Medicare Payment for Coronavirus Lab
Tests," MedTech Dive, April 15, 2020, https://www.medtechdive.com/news
/cms-doubles-medicare-payment-for-coronavirus-lab-tests/576120.

47. "Global Partnership to Make Available 120 Million Affordable, Quality
COVID-19 Rapid Tests for Low- and Middle-Income Countries," press release, World Health Organization, September 28, 2020, https://www.who
.int/news/item/28-09-2020-global-partnership-to-make-available-120
-million-affordable-quality-covid-19-rapid-tests-for-low--and-middle-income
-countries; "How We're Doing It Wrong and How to Fix It, with Rajiv Shah,"
In the Bubble with Andy Slavitt, accessed October 14, 2020, https://www

.lemonadamedia.com/podcast/how-were-doing-it-wrong-and-how-to-fix-it
-with-rajiv-shah.

48. Paul Fronstin and Stephen A. Woodbury, "How Many Americans Have Lost
Jobs with Employer Health Coverage During the Pandemic?," Commonwealth
Fund, October 7, 2020, https://doi.org/10.26099/q9p1-tz63; Reed Abelson,
"Major U.S. Health Insurers Report Big Profits, Benefiting from the Pandemic,"
New York Times, August 5, 2020, https://www.nytimes.com/2020/08/05/health
/covid-insurance-profits.html; Minemyer, "Health Insurers' Profits Topped $35B
Last Year. Medicare Advantage Is the Common Thread."

49. Gretchen Morgenson, Rich Gardella, and Andrew W. Lehren, "Firms with
Trump Links or Worth $100 Million Got Small Business Loans," NBC News,
April 24, 2020, https://www.nbcnews.com/business/economy/firms-trump
-links-or-worth-100-million-got-small-business-n1190741.

50. Theodoric Meyer and Adam Cancryn, "Chris Christie Cashes In on Coronavirus Lobbying," *Politico*, July 23, 2020, https://www.politico.com/news/2020
/07/23/chris-christie-cashes-in-on-coronavirus-lobbying-380640?cid=covid_m.

51. "The Top 15 Medical Device Companies in the World in 2020," Get-
Reskilled, last updated May 2020, https://www.getreskilled.com/medical
-device-companies; Geraldine Grones, "Top 10 Health Insurance Companies in the US," *Insurance Business*, February 3, 2020, https://www
.insurancebusinessmag.com/us/news/healthcare/top-10-health-insurance
-companies-in-the-us-212292.aspx; Maia Anderson, "Top 10 Pharma Companies by Revenue," *Becker's Hospital Review*, March 4, 2020, https://www
.beckershospitalreview.com/pharmacy/top-10-pharma-companies-by
-revenue.html; "50 Top-Grossing For-Profit Hospitals."

Chapter 10: Anti-Expert, Pro-Magic

1. Kiera Butler, "The US Has Reached the Grim Milestone of 200,000 COVID-19
Deaths. We Could Have Avoided It," *Mother Jones*, September 19, 2020,
https://www.motherjones.com/politics/2020/09/200000-coronavirus-deaths
-experts-done-differently.

2. World Health Organization, "Measles," accessed October 14, 2020, https://www
.who.int/news-room/fact-sheets/detail/measles; Michael Skapinker, "Why Rich
Countries Are More Prone to 'Vaccine Hesitancy,'" *Financial Times*, June 25,
2019, https://www.ft.com/content/2271a90c-942d-11e9-b7ea-60e35ef678d2;
Lena H. Sun, "Percentage of Young U.S. Children Who Don't Receive Any
Vaccines Has Quadrupled Since 2001," *Washington Post*, October 11, 2018,
https://www.washingtonpost.com/national/health-science/percentage-of
-young-us-children-who-dont-receive-any-vaccines-has-quadrupled-since
-2001/2018/10/11/4a9cca98-cd0d-11e8-920f-dd52e1ae4570_story.html;

Fiona M. Guerra et al., "The Basic Reproduction Number (R0) of Measles: A Systematic Review," *Lancet Infectious Diseases* 17, no. 12 (July 27, 2017): e420–28, https://doi.org/10.1016/s1473-3099(17)30307-9.

3. Olivia Messer, "The Terrifying Reality of Trump's Coronavirus Promise," *Daily Beast*, February 25, 2020, https://www.thedailybeast.com/trump-hints -coronavirus-vaccine-is-very-close-heres-the-scarier-reality.

4. Mike Pence, "There Isn't a Coronavirus 'Second Wave,'" *Wall Street Journal*, June 16, 2020, https://www.wsj.com/articles/there-isnt-a-coronavirus-second -wave-11592327890; Louise Hall, "Pence Thinks a Miracle Is 'Around the Corner' for Coronavirus Pandemic," *Independent*, August 22, 2020, https:// www.independent.co.uk/news/world/americas/us-politics/coronavirus-pence -biden-covid-cure-vaccine-trump-2020-election-a9682256.html.

5. Gregg Gonsalves and Forrest Crawford, "How Mike Pence Made Indiana's HIV Outbreak Worse," *Politico*, March 2, 2020, https://www.politico.com /news/magazine/2020/03/02/how-mike-pence-made-indianas-hiv-outbreak -worse-118648; Jason Silverstein, "Mike Pence Said Smoking 'Doesn't Kill' and Faced Criticism for His Response to HIV. Now He's Leading the Coronavirus Response," CBS News, February 29, 2020, https://www .cbsnews.com/news/coronavirus-mike-pence-health-science-smoking-hiv; Feliks Garcia, "Mike Pence Once Said Condoms Are 'Very Poor' Defence Against STDs," *Independent*, July 21, 2016, https://www.independent .co.uk/news/world/americas/us-politics/mike-pence-condoms-very-poor -protection-stds-policies-2002-a7149106.html; Ryan Schleeter, "5 Real Things Mike Pence Has Said About Climate Change," Greenpeace USA, July 15, 2016, https://www.greenpeace.org/usa/5-real-things-mike-pence-has-said-about -climate-change.

6. "How Will COVID-19 End? With Ed Yong," *In the Bubble with Andy Slavitt*, September 21, 2020, https://www.lemonadamedia.com/podcast/how-will -covid19-end-with-ed-yong.

7. "Vaccine Safety Questions and Answers," Center for Biologics Evaluation and Research, FDA, April 5, 2019, https://www.fda.gov/vaccines-blood -biologics/safety-availability-biologics/vaccine-safety-questions-and-answers; "The FDA Science Forum," Office of the Commissioner, FDA, September 23, 2019, https://www.fda.gov/science-research/about-science-research-fda/fda -science-forum.

8. Dan Levine and Marisa Taylor, "Exclusive: Top FDA Official Says Would Resign if Agency Rubber-Stamps an Unproven COVID-19 Vaccine," Reuters, August 20, 2020, https://www.reuters.com/article/us-health-coronavirus -vaccines-fda-exclu/exclusive-top-fda-official-says-would-resign-if-agency -rubber-stamps-an-unproven-covid-19-vaccine-idUSKBN25H03H.

9. Scott Detrow, "Trump Dismisses Top Scientist Rick Bright as 'Disgruntled Employee,'" NPR, May 6, 2020, https://www.npr.org/sections/coronavirus -live-updates/2020/05/06/851719205/trump-dismisses-top-scientist-rick -bright-as-disgruntled-employee.

10. Elon Musk, "Maybe worth considering chloroquine for C19," Twitter, March 16, 2020, 4:31 p.m., https://twitter.com/elonmusk/status/1239650597906898947.

11. Will Stone, "Government Scientist Adds to Whistle-Blower Complaint and Quits NIH," NPR, October 6, 2020, https://www.npr.org/sections/coronavirus -live-updates/2020/10/06/920985099/government-scientist-tops-up-whistle -blower-complaint-and-quits-nih.

12. Andrew Solender, "All the Times Trump Has Promoted Hydroxychloroquine," *Forbes*, May 22, 2020, https://www.forbes.com/sites/andrewsolender/2020 /05/22/all-the-times-trump-promoted-hydroxychloroquine; Rick Bright, "Request for Emergency Use Authorization for Use of Chloroquine Phosphate or Hydroxychloroquine Sulfate Supplied from the Strategic National Stockpile for Treatment of 2019 Coronavirus Disease," March 28, 2020.

13. Saleha Mohsin and Josh Wingrove, "Trump Says FDA May Be Delaying Plasma Approval over Politics," Bloomberg, August 19, 2020, https://www .bloomberg.com/news/articles/2020-08-19/trump-says-fda-may-be-delaying -plasma-approval-over-politics; Donald J. Trump, "The deep state, or whoever, over at the FDA is making it very difficult for drug companies to get people in order to test the vaccines and therapeutics. Obviously, they are hoping to delay the answer until after November 3rd. Must focus on speed, and saving lives! @SteveFDA," Twitter, August 22, 2020, 7:49 p.m., https://twitter.com /realDonaldTrump/status/1297138862108663808; Aaron Blake, "FDA Commissioner Stephen Hahn Echoes Trump's Hyperbole on Plasma," *Washington Post*, August 25, 2020, https://www.washingtonpost.com/politics/2020/08/24 /fda-head-toes-trump-line-plasma-goes-too-far.

14. Michael J. Joyner et al., "Effect of Convalescent Plasma on Mortality Among Hospitalized Patients with COVID-19: Initial Three-Month Experience," MedRxiv, August 12, 2020, https://doi.org/10.1101/2020.08.12.20169359.

15. Andy Slavitt, "FDA Chief Apologizes for COVID-19 Plasma Exaggeration—But Trump's Endgame Is Clear," NBC News, August 31, 2020, https://www.nbcnews .com/think/opinion/fda-chief-apologizes-covid-19-plasma-exaggeration-trump -s-endgame-ncna1238721.

16. Transcript, *CNN Tonight*, CNN, September 22, 2020, http://transcripts.cnn .com/TRANSCRIPTS/2009/22/cnnt.02.html.

17. Jeff Mason, "Trump Says May Block Stricter FDA Guidelines for COVID-19 Vaccine," Reuters, September 24, 2020, https://www.reuters.com/article/us -health-coronavirus-usa-vaccine-trump-idUSKCN26E3M5.

18. "Open Letter to Stephen Hahn Regarding a Vaccine," August 5, 2020, https://cspinet.org/sites/default/files/COVID_Vaccine_Letter_to_FDA_8.5.2020.pdf.

19. Adam Cancryn and Dan Diamond, "An Angry Azar Floats Plans to Oust FDA's Hahn," *Politico*, October 22, 2020, https://www.politico.com/news/2020/10/22/azar-plans-oust-hahn-fda-431139.

20. Sheila Kaplan, "In 'Power Grab,' Health Secretary Azar Asserts Authority over F.D.A.," *New York Times*, September 19, 2020, https://www.nytimes.com/2020/09/19/health/azar-hhs-fda.html.

21. Dan Diamond, "Trump Officials Interfered with CDC Reports on Covid-19," *Politico*, September 11, 2020, https://www.politico.com/news/2020/09/11/exclusive-trump-officials-interfered-with-cdc-reports-on-covid-19–412809; Dan Diamond, Adam Cancryn, and Sarah Owermohle, "'It Just Created a Public Relations Nightmare': Inside Michael Caputo's Time at HHS," *Politico*, September 16, 2020, https://www.politico.com/news/2020/09/16/how-michael-caputo-shook-up-hhs-416632.

22. Gino Spocchia, "Video Emerges Showing Trump Talking About Cutting Pandemic Team in 2018, Despite Saying Last Week 'I Didn't Know About It,'" *Independent*, March 16, 2020, https://www.independent.co.uk/news/world/americas/us-politics/coronavirus-video-trump-pandemic-team-cut-2018-a9405191.html.

23. Nick Gass, "Trump: 'The Experts Are Terrible,'" *Politico*, April 4, 2016, https://www.politico.com/blogs/2016-gop-primary-live-updates-and-results/2016/04/donald-trump-foreign-policy-experts-221528.

24. Haley Britzky, "Everything Trump Says He Knows 'More About Than Anybody,'" *Axios*, January 5, 2019, https://www.axios.com/everything-trump-says-he-knows-more-about-than-anybody-b278b592-cff0-47dc-a75f-5767f42bcf1e.html.

25. Andy Slavitt, "The CDC website says that only 6 percent of the people who have died from COVID actually died of COVID because they also had other conditions. Social media is promoting this to minimize COVID. This political spin doesn't prevent disease. It causes it," Twitter, August 30, 2020, 11:51 a.m., https://twitter.com/ASlavitt/status/1300098832605286401.

26. "What No One Knows About COVID-19, with Larry Brilliant," *In the Bubble with Andy Slavitt*, July 22, 2020, https://www.lemonadamedia.com/podcast/what-no-one-knows-about-covid-19-with-larry-brilliant.

27. "What No One Knows About COVID-19, with Larry Brilliant."

28. "Mini-Episode: Living Through Two Public Health Crises, with Dr. Leana Wen," *In the Bubble with Andy Slavitt*, June 8, 2020, https://www.lemonadamedia.com/podcast/mini-episode-living-through-two-public-health-crises-with-leana-wen.

29. "Mark D. Smith, Former CEO, California HealthCare Foundation," Voices in Leadership, Harvard T. H. Chan School of Public Health, accessed October 15, 2020, https://www.hsph.harvard.edu/voices/events/smith.

30. Patricia Goodson, "Questioning the HIV-AIDS Hypothesis: 30 Years of Dissent," *Frontiers in Public Health* 2 (September 23, 2014): 154, https://www.ncbi.nlm.nih.gov/pmc/articles/PMC4172096, doi: 10.3389/fpubh.2014.00154.

31. Samantha Cole, "Quote of the Week: Double Your Failure Rate," *Fast Company*, July 14, 2014, https://www.fastcompany.com/3033003/quote-of-the-week-double-your-failure-rate.

32. "How Will COVID-19 End? With Ed Yong."

33. "Mini-Episode: The Pandemic Broke Our Brains, with Chris Hayes," *In the Bubble with Andy Slavitt*, October 7, 2020, https://www.lemonadamedia.com/podcast/in-the-bubble-chris-hayes.

34. Andy Slavitt, "We have former newspaper reporters explaining epidemiology and the natural history of disease," Twitter, August 8, 2020, 7:48 p.m., https://twitter.com/ASlavitt/status/1292246399720083456.

35. "Anthony Fauci Has Been Wrong About Everything I Have Interacted with Him On: Peter Navarro," *USA Today*, July 14, 2020, https://www.usatoday.com/story/opinion/todaysdebate/2020/07/14/anthony-fauci-wrong-with-me-peter-navarro-editorials-debates/5439374002.

36. "See Dr. Anthony Fauci's Heated Exchange with Jim Jordan over Protests During Coronavirus," YouTube, posted by CNN, July 31, 2020, https://www.youtube.com/watch?v=oSCSWVrcCtA.

37. "Can We Still Trust the CDC? With Tom Frieden," *In the Bubble with Andy Slavitt*, accessed October 15, 2020, https://www.lemonadamedia.com/podcast/can-we-still-trust-the-cdc-with-tom-frieden.

38. Ramsey Touchberry, "Secret White House Coronavirus Task Force Reports Contradict Public Claims by Trump, Pence," *Newsweek*, August 31, 2020, https://www.newsweek.com/secret-white-house-coronavirus-task-force-reports-contradict-public-claims-trump-pence-1528741.

39. Nathaniel Weixel, "Private Coronavirus Task Force Reports Warned States of Virus Spread," *The Hill*, August 31, 2020, https://thehill.com/policy/healthcare/514468-private-coronavirus-task-force-reports-warn-states-of-virus-spread; Pence, "There Isn't a Coronavirus 'Second Wave'"; "Select Subcommittee Releases Eight Weeks of Coronavirus Task Force Reports Kept Secret by the White House," House Select Subcommittee on the Coronavirus Crisis, August 31, 2020, https://coronavirus.house.gov/news/press-releases/select-subcommittee-releases-eight-weeks-coronavirus-task-force-reports-kept; Justine Coleman, "Trump Breaks with Fauci: US in 'Good Place' in Fight Against Virus," *The Hill*, July 7, 2020, https://thehill.com/homenews

/administration/506307-trump-breaks-with-fauci-us-in-good-place-in-fight
-against-virus.

40. Andy Slavitt, "When all opinions are equal, hierarchy decides right from wrong," Twitter, August 8, 2020, https://twitter.com/aslavitt/status /1292246422226710529?lang=en.

41. Kevin Breuninger, "Trump Attacks Dr. Birx After She Said U.S. Reached 'New Phase' in Coronavirus Fight," CNBC, August 3, 2020, https://www.cnbc.com /2020/08/03/trump-attacks-dr-birx-after-she-said-us-reached-new-phase-in -coronavirus-fight.html.

42. Sanjay Gupta, "New WH Adviser Pushes Controversial Pandemic Response," *Anderson Cooper 360*, CNN, September 2, 2020, https://www.cnn.com /videos/health/2020/09/02/sanjay-gupta-herd-immunity-wh-adviser-ac360 -pkg-vpx.cnn.

43. Kaitlan Collins, "Trump Adds Coronavirus Adviser Who Echoes His Un-scientific Claims," CNN, August 12, 2020, https://www.cnn.com/2020/08 /12/politics/scott-atlas-donald-trump-coronavirus/index.html; Kiran Stacey, "Trump Covid Adviser Scott Atlas Pushes Herd Immunity," *Financial Times*, October 25, 2020, https://www.ft.com/content/9c95268e-5a65-48c4-bbaa -a4d88c4b5c03.

44. Lucien Brueggeman and Libbey Cathey, "Former Stanford Colleagues Warn Dr. Scott Atlas Fosters 'Falsehoods and Misrepresentations of Science,'" ABC News, September 10, 2020, https://abcnews.go.com/Politics/stanford-colleagues-warn -dr-scott-atlas-fosters-falsehoods/story?id=72926212.

45. Andy Slavitt, "How Trump Plans to Discredit Health Experts and Play Politics with a Crisis," Medium Coronavirus Blog, May 8, 2020, https:// coronavirus.medium.com/how-trump-plans-to-discredit-health-experts-and -play-politics-with-a-crisis-7588b4f6b13c.

Chapter 11: Deniers, Fauxers, and Herders (Oh My)

1. "Tucker Carlson: There's No Evidence Coronavirus Lockdowns Saved Lives. Mass Quarantines May Have Killed People," Fox News, May 22, 2020, https:// www.foxnews.com/opinion/tucker-carlson-theres-no-evidence-coronavirus -lockdowns-saved-lives-mass-quarantines-may-have-killed-people.

2. COVID Tracking Project, "Our Data," accessed September 27, 2020, https:// covidtracking.com/data.

3. COVID Tracking Project, "Our Data."

4. COVID Tracking Project, "Our Data"; Molly Gamble, "States Ranked by COVID-19 Test Positivity Rates: Nov. 3," *Becker's Hospital Review*, accessed November 4, 2020, https://www.beckershospitalreview.com/public-health/states -ranked-by-covid-19-test-positivity-rates-july-14.html.

5. Katherine J. Wu, "Covid Combat Fatigue: 'I Would Come Home with Tears in My Eyes,'" *New York Times*, November 25, 2020, https://www.nytimes.com /2020/11/25/health/doctors-nurses-covid-stress.html.

6. Mary Van Beusekom, "Stop Attacking Public Health Officials, Experts Plead," Center for Infectious Disease Research and Policy, University of Minnesota, August 6, 2020, https://www.cidrap.umn.edu/news-perspective/2020 /08/stop-attacking-public-health-officials-experts-plead; "Toolkit: Everything You Need to Know About Vaccines," *In the Bubble with Andy Slavitt*, July 13, 2020, https://www.lemonadamedia.com/podcast/toolkit-everything-you -need-to-know-about-vaccines; Mike Stunson, "Fauci Says on CNN Podcast He Now Has Personal Security," *Miami Herald*, July 24, 2020, https://www .miamiherald.com/news/coronavirus/article244460877.html.

7. Emily Badger and Kevin Quealy, "Red vs. Blue on Coronavirus Concern: The Gap Is Still Big but Closing," *New York Times*, March 21, 2020, https:// www.nytimes.com/interactive/2020/03/21/upshot/coronavirus-public-opinion .html.

8. Lloyd Doggett, "Timeline of Trump's Coronavirus Responses," https://doggett .house.gov/media-center/blog-posts/timeline-trump-s-coronavirus -responses.

9. Andy Slavitt, "Trump's defenders like to say 'It wouldn't have been any different under Obama.' It would have been different under anyone but a madman," Twitter, September 9, 2020, 6:15 p.m., https://twitter.com/ASlavitt/status /1303819438437920771.

10. Andy Slavitt, "They need surrogates I guess because there's only so many ways to say 'it's ok for some people to die' without sounding like an asshole," Twitter, May 8, 2020, 9:12 p.m., https://twitter.com/ASlavitt/status /1258927871634145281.

11. Senator Scott Jensen, "Flu vs. COVID-19," Facebook Watch, March 27, 2020, https://www.facebook.com/watch/?v=616887239159067; Michelle Rogers, "Fact Check: Hospitals Get Paid More if Patients Listed as COVID-19, on Ventilators," *The Star* (Port St. Joe, FL), April 25, 2020, https://www.starfl .com/news/20200425/fact-check-hospitals-get-paid-more-if-patients-listed-as -covid-19-on-ventilators.

12. Scott Jensen, "Conversation About COVID-19," livestreamed event on Facebook, March 29, 2020, https://www.facebook.com/1492673654369368 /videos/549373252369714/?__so__=channel_tab&__rv__=all_videos_card.

13. "Immunizing the Public Against Misinformation," World Health Organization, August 25, 2020, https://www.who.int/news-room/feature-stories/detail /immunizing-the-public-against-misinformation.

14. Sheryl Gay Stolberg and Noah Weiland, "Study Finds 'Single Largest Driver' of Coronavirus Misinformation: Trump," *New York Times*, September 30,

2020, https://www.nytimes.com/2020/09/30/us/politics/trump-coronavirus
-misinformation.html; Sheera Frenkel, Ben Decker, and Davey Alba, "How
the 'Plandemic' Movie and Its Falsehoods Spread Widely Online," *New York
Times*, May 20, 2020, https://www.nytimes.com/2020/05/20/technology
/plandemic-movie-youtube-facebook-coronavirus.html.

15. Tim Walker, "Trump Says COVID-19 Could Be Stopped by 'Herd Mentality,'" *Guardian*, September 16, 2020, https://www.theguardian.com/us-news
/2020/sep/16/first-thing-trump-says-covid-19-could-be-stopped-by-herd
-mentality.

16. "Herd Immunity and COVID-19 (Coronavirus): What You Need to Know,"
Mayo Clinic, June 6, 2020, https://www.mayoclinic.org/diseases-conditions
/coronavirus/in-depth/herd-immunity-and-coronavirus/art-20486808.

17. "National Coronavirus Response: A Road Map to Reopening," American Enterprise Institute, March 29, 2020, https://www.aei.org/research
-products/report/national-coronavirus-response-a-road-map-to-reopening;
"Great Barrington Declaration and Petition," October 4, 2020, https://
gbdeclaration.org.

18. Joel Achenbach, "Proposal to Hasten Herd Immunity Grabs White House
Attention, Appalls Top Scientists," *Anchorage Daily News*, October 13, 2020,
https://www.adn.com/nation-world/2020/10/13/proposal-to-hasten-herd
-immunity-grabs-white-house-attention-appalls-top-scientists.

19. "COVIDView, Key Updates for Week 22," Centers for Disease Control and
Prevention, June 5, 2020, https://www.cdc.gov/coronavirus/2019-ncov/covid
-data/covidview/past-reports/06052020.html.

20. COVID Tracking Project, "Our Data."

21. Debbie Cenziper, Joel Jacobs, and Shawn Mulcahy, "As Pandemic Raged and
Thousands Died, Government Regulators Cleared Most Nursing Homes of
Infection-Control Violations," *Washington Post*, October 29, 2020, https://
www.washingtonpost.com/business/2020/10/29/nursing-home-deaths-fines;
"COVID-19 Nursing Home Dataset," Centers for Medicare and Medicaid Ser-
vices, November 19, 2020, https://data.cms.gov/Special-Programs-Initiatives
-COVID-19-Nursing-Home/COVID-19-Nursing-Home-Dataset/s2uc-8wxp;
Robert King, "KFF: More Than 100k Died in Nursing Homes, Long-Term
Care Facilities from COVID-19," Fierce Healthcare, November 25, 2020,
https://www.fiercehealthcare.com/hospitals/kff-more-than-100k-died-nursing
-homes-long-term-care-facilities-from-covid-19#.

22. Suzi Ring and Jason Gale, "Can You Get Covid Twice? What Reinfection
Cases Really Mean," *Washington Post*, October 28, 2020, https://www
.washingtonpost.com/business/can-you-get-covid-twice-what-reinfection
-cases-really-mean/2020/10/28/1cd3b53a-18d9-11eb-8bda-814ca56e138b
_story.html.

23. Andy Slavitt, "We have learned the daunting power of exponential math when it comes to infection rate or R0. At an R0 of 2.3, 1 person spreads COVID-19 to an average of 4100 people in 10 generations. At 1.3, it's only 14. At 3.3 it's 153,000 people. But what if you reverse that," Twitter, April 25, 2020, 11:11 p.m., https://twitter.com/ASlavitt/status/1254246666686922752. Lightly edited for use here.

24. Xiaojian Xie et al., "Exhaled Droplets Due to Talking and Coughing," *Interface Focus* 6, suppl. 6 (December 6, 2009): S703–14, https://doi.org/10.1098/rsif.2009.0388.focus; Jeremy Howard et al., "Face Masks Against COVID-19: An Evidence Review," preprint, April 10, 2020, https://files.fast.ai/papers/masks_lit_review.pdf; "NIOSH-Approved Particulate Filtering Facepiece Respirators," Centers for Disease Control, last reviewed April 9, 2020, https://www.cdc.gov/niosh/npptl/topics/respirators/disp_part/default.html.

25. Shuo Feng et al., "Rational Use of Face Masks in the COVID-19 Pandemic," *Lancet Respiratory Medicine* 8, no. 5 (May 1, 2020): 434–36, https://www.thelancet.com/journals/lanres/article/PIIS2213-2600(20)30134-X/fulltext?fbclid=IwAR13Xz-m-mUi-8g1O01FREbSEjl3tUxpSBiNqXufxqSaIXo0QV_cyWu3Qx4; Wei Lyu and George L. Wehby, "Community Use of Face Masks and COVID-19: Evidence from a Natural Experiment of State Mandates in the US," *Health Affairs* 39, no. 8 (June 16, 2020), https://www.healthaffairs.org/doi/10.1377/hlthaff.2020.00818; Christopher Leffler et al., "Association of Country-Wide Coronavirus Mortality with Demographics, Testing, Lockdowns, and Public Wearing of Masks (Update June 15, 2020)," MedRxiv, June 15, 2020, https://www.medrxiv.org/content/10.1101/2020.05.22.20109231v3?versioned=true; Apoorva Mandavilli, "The Price for Not Wearing Masks: Perhaps 130,000 Lives," *New York Times*, last updated October 30, 2020, https://www.nytimes.com/2020/10/23/health/covid-deaths.html; IHME Covid-19 Forecasting Team, "Modeling COVID-19 Scenarios for the United States," *Nature Medicine*, October 23, 2020, https://www.nature.com/articles/s41591-020-1132-9.

26. "CDC Director Robert Redfield Coronavirus Response Senate Hearing Transcript," September 16, 2020, https://www.rev.com/blog/transcripts/cdc-coronavirus-response-senate-hearing-transcript-september-16.

27. Andy Slavitt, "Science Is Needed to Rescue the Nation from COVID-19, but Not Just Traditional Biomedical Science," *JAMA Network*, October 8, 2020, https://jamanetwork.com/channels/health-forum/fullarticle/2771804.

28. Dawn Baumgartner Vaughan, "NC GOP Governor Candidate Dan Forest Wants to End Masks Rule," *Raleigh News and Observer*, updated September 17, 2020, https://www.newsobserver.com/news/politics-government/election/article245779135.html; Associated Press, "'I'll Kiss Everyone': Trump Claims He Has Immunity at First Rally Since Covid Diagnosis—Video," *Guardian*, October 12, 2020, https://www.theguardian.com/global/video

/2020/oct/12/ill-kiss-everyone-trump-claims-he-has-immunity-at-first-rally
-since-covid-diagnosis-video.

29. Jane Onyanga-Omara, Ryan W. Miller, Joshua Bote, and Grace Hauck, "Donald, Melania Trump COVID Positive, Biden Negative: What We Know," *USA Today*, updated October 3, 2020, https://www.usatoday.com /story/news/nation/2020/10/02/president-trump-tests-positive-covid-19 -heres-what-we-know/5892425002; Maggie Haberman and Michael D. Shear, "Trump Says He'll Begin 'Quarantine Process' After Hope Hicks Tests Positive for Coronavirus," *New York Times*, October 1, 2020, https:// www.nytimes.com/2020/10/01/us/politics/hope-hicks-coronavirus.html; Jennifer Steinhauer, "Trump Suggests Gold Star Families May Be to Blame for His Infection," *New York Times*, October 8, 2020, https://www.nytimes .com/2020/10/08/us/politics/trump-coronavirus-gold-star-families.html; Ben Kamisar and Melissa Holzberg, "Poll: Majority Still Fears Virus Exposure as Trump Says Not to Be 'Afraid,'" NBC News, October 6, 2020, https://www.nbcnews.com/politics/2020-election/poll-majority-still-fears -virus-exposure-trump-says-not-be-n1242195; Christina Morales, Allyson Waller, and Marie Fazio, "A Timeline of Trump's Symptoms and Treatments," *New York Times*, October 14, 2020, https://www.nytimes.com /2020/10/04/us/trump-covid-symptoms-timeline.html.

30. John Haltiwanger, "Trump's Car Ride That Put Secret Service Agents at Risk Was Reportedly a Compromise After Doctors Refused to Discharge Him from the Hospital," *Business Insider*, October 5, 2020, https://www.businessinsider.com /trump-covid-19-car-ride-compromise-after-demanded-leave-hospital-2020-10.

31. Hannah Miao, "More Than 130 Secret Service Officers Are Isolating Due to Covid-19 Outbreak, Report Says," CNBC, November 13, 2020, https://www .cnbc.com/2020/11/13/more-than-130-secret-service-officers-are-isolating -due-to-covid-19-outbreak-report-says.html.

32. "COVID-19 at the White House—Contact Tracking," Tableau Software, accessedNovember3,2020,https://public.tableau.com/views/COVID-19attheWhite House-ContactTracking/ByEvent? percent3Aembed=y& percent3Ashow VizHome=no&percent3Adisplay_count=y&percent3Adisplay_static_image =y&percent3AbootstrapWhenNotified=true&percent3Alanguage=en&:embed =y&:showVizHome=n&:apiID=host0#navType=0&navSrc=Parse.

33. "I Got COVID-19 from the White House (with Michael Shear)," *In the Bubble with Andy Slavitt*, October 28, 2020, https://podcasts.apple.com/us/podcast /i-got-covid-19-from-the-white-house-with-michael-shear/id1504128553?i =1000496327228.

34. Zamira Rahim, "Boris Johnson Warns Against Relaxing UK Lockdown as He Returns to Work Following Illness," CNN, April 27, 2020, https://www

.cnn.com/2020/04/27/uk/boris-johnson-downing-street-speech-return-intl
-gbr/index.html.

35. Katherine J. Wu, "The Coronavirus Has Claimed 2.5 Million Years of Potential Life in the U.S., Study Finds," *New York Times*, October 21, 2020, https://
www.nytimes.com/2020/10/21/health/coronavirus-statistics-deaths.html.

36. Bryce Covert, "How Medicaid Expansion Is Transforming Politics as We Know It," *The Nation*, December 16, 2019, https://www.thenation.com/article
/archive/kentucky-medicaid-expansion-voter-turnout.

37. "The Governor with the Secret Formula on COVID (with Governor Andy Beshear)," *In the Bubble with Andy Slavitt*, September 14, 2020, https://www
.lemonadamedia.com/podcast/the-governor-with-the-secret-formula-on-covid
-with-governor-andy-beshear.

38. "List of Countries by Total Wealth," Wikipedia, accessed November 6, 2020, https://en.wikipedia.org/wiki/List_of_countries_by_total_wealth#cite_note
-CS_2019-1-3.

39. "The Governor with the Secret Formula on COVID."

Chapter 12: The Work to Do

1. The COVID Tracking Project, https://covidtracking.com/data.

2. Steven Aftergood, "The History of the Soviet Biological Weapons Program," Federation of American Scientists, July 18, 2012, https://fas.org/blogs/secrecy
/2012/07/soviet_bw.

3. Kayla Chadwick, "I Don't Know How to Explain to You That You Should Care About Other People," *HuffPost*, June 26, 2017, https://www.huffpost
.com/entry/i-dont-know-how-to-explain-to-you-that-you-should_b
_59519811e4b0f078efd98440.

4. Dan Hodges, "In retrospect Sandy Hook marked the end of the US gun control debate. Once America decided killing children was bearable, it was over," Twitter, June 19, 2015, 1:07 p.m., https://twitter.com/DPJHodges
/status/611943312401002496; Joanna Walters, "Trump Twists Stats on Police Brutality: 'More White People' Are Killed," *Guardian*, July 15, 2020, https://www.theguardian.com/us-news/2020/jul/14/donald-trump-george
-floyd-police-killings; "11 Facts About Hunger in the US," DoSomething
.org, accessed October 30, 2020, https://www.dosomething.org/us/facts/11
-facts-about-hunger-us; "Poll: Nearly 1 in 4 Americans Taking Prescription Drugs Say It's Difficult to Afford Their Medicines, Including Larger Shares Among Those with Health Issues, with Low Incomes and Nearing Medicare Age," KFF, March 1, 2019, https://www.kff.org/health-costs/press-release/poll
-nearly-1-in-4-americans-taking-prescription-drugs-say-its-difficult-to-afford
-medicines-including-larger-shares-with-low-incomes/.

5. "Drug Overdose Deaths," Centers for Disease Control, March 19, 2020, https://www.cdc.gov/drugoverdose/data/statedeaths.html; "Suicide," National Institute of Mental Health, accessed October 27, 2020, https://www.nimh.nih.gov/health/statistics/suicide.shtml.

6. Edgar Allan Poe, "The Masque of the Red Death," accessed October 30, 2020, https://www.poemuseum.org/the-masque-of-the-red-death.

Afterword

1. John Bacon, Jorge L. Ortiz, and Doyle Rice, "Coronavirus Live Updates: As US Death Toll Approaches 400K, New Variants Threaten to Add to Struggle; Americans' Trust in Vaccines Grows," *USA Today*, January 18, 2021, https://www.usatoday.com/story/news/health/2021/01/18/covid-updates-vaccinations-lag-death-toll-approaches-400-000/4201783001/.

INDEX